Nice to a Fault?

Redefining Kindness in Marriage

CAROLYN KLASSEN

DEDICATION

To my husband. Jim puts in deliberate effort every day to keep our
marriage alive and vital. While books and teachers and colleagues
have taught me about marriage, you give me the incredible
experience of knowing what an engaged and loving husband feels
like—every day.

CONTENTS

ACKNOWLEDGMENTS

To the clients—husbands and wives—who have taught me about relationships, courage, fear and vulnerability. Counseling school taught me some. You taught me *much* more. Even as we were exploring your story, your questions, your pain, your relationships, and your journey, I was learning from you. I am grateful.

Carolyn Klassen

PROLOGUE

I've been a therapist for a lot of years, with men, women, and couples. So often, even when I work with individuals, I hear people are doing the best they can, but it falls short of being able to meaningfully connect in the most important relationship in their lives: their marriage.

Our Western world raises boys and girls in ways that make marriages difficult when they grow up. It might be the twenty-first century, but gender stereotypes persist, often in quiet and subtle ways. We'd like to think we are long past this stuff. We are not. In the quietness of the counseling office, I hear how destructive gender norms are alive and not so well. Women are acculturated to be quiet, cooperative and "nice". Nice so often gets in the way of kind. We instruct men to be tough, work hard, and not be seen as tender. When couples get locked into who our culture tells them to be, it takes away from being who they really are. It takes away from being able to authentically connect.

Our world, as we know it, makes it harder to have a vital and enriching marriage good for both partners.

May the pages you read inside this book challenge some of those patterns in which you and your partner find yourselves stuck. May these pages open doors to tender conversations that can bring back some closeness you both want. May reading spur challenging but good conversations that will get you, as a couple, to grow. If it means walking into a therapist's office where you can both do the hard work of finding your way back to each other, I hope this book inspires you to do that. Formerly, this book was titled, *My Marriage is Almost Dead and My Husband Doesn't Get it.* But the truth is, this book was always for a broader audience of wives looking to improve their marriage with a great guy who hasn't always been a great husband. Chapters have been added. This book is for all wives who wonder if there isn't something more.

As a therapist, I'm all about better relationships. I'm all about helping people in my office, through the written word, and in the seminars and workshops I deliver, to connect better with each other. The hardest relationships are also usually the ones that are the most important. Marriage is a super important relationship. Divorce is excruciatingly painful for the couple, their children, family, and friends.

But, as a therapist, I am not about saving marriages at all cost. This book is not intended to minimize abuse of any kind. This book is not encouraging you to stay in an unsafe home. Or intended to have women who have been made to feel small in their lives feel any smaller. This is about strengthening and empowering you as a woman to speak truth in a way your husband will receive it.

If you have been beaten down, physically and/or mentally and/or emotionally, know you may need extra help to actually become empowered. No one deserves to be hurt—and that includes you. Please ensure that you are safe. Don't use this book to feel worse about yourself, please.

Now—on to finding words and language to understand how you feel...which will shape how you talk...which will impact on your behaviors and actions…which will shape your life. May this book shape your life positively because of the time spent pondering these pages.

1 BE KIND: "NICE DOESN'T WORK FOR ANYBODY

It breaks my heart when women are so nice that they don't tell their partners or their friends or their kids when they are mad. When women are hurting, or feeling ignored or upset, or things just aren't working, culture often dictates they swallow their discomfort.

It frustrates me when women:

- suppress what they want to have happen
- pretend it didn't hurt all that much, or
- stop themselves from expressing a different opinion on the matter

It particularly drives me a little crazy when women are doing all of these nice things for the sake of the relationship.

- Isn't it nice to let him choose pizza without mentioning you'd really prefer sushi? Haven't you been taught the "right thing" to give in when he says he wants pizza without working out a collaborative solution for how to make it work for both of you?

- Isn't it thoughtful to pick up his socks over and over (and over and over) saying nothing? Or if you say something, and he doesn't listen, then giving up and just doing it, anyway? (And then, nice is pretending that the growing resentment isn't really there!)
- Isn't it polite to not belabor how painful it was at the party when he got drunk and was rude to your friends? Not bringing it up the next day makes the whole day go so much easier! (Even though you're still stewing about it.)
- Doesn't it help the relationship to "suck it up" when he trivializes the promotion you got at work and goes on as if it doesn't matter? After all, women are supposed to not need the encouragement of their spouses these days (or so goes the feminist line, anyway).

What breaks my heart is that well intentioned, lovely, sensitive, caring women live the above, while:

- swallowing hurts,
- pretending they don't have preferences,
- ignoring their own sensitivities
- trying their darndest to express them so caringly to the other—that they end up dismissed/ignored or not heard at all

What frustrates me is the cost of the months and years and decades of a wife suppressing her own preferences and ideas, being hurt repeatedly with no change on behalf of the other. Frankly, it *wears on a woman*. It then *wears on the relationship*, and the rope of connection becomes increasingly frayed...

...more and more...

until, one day...

it snaps.

And. She's. Done.

She has **niced** the connection right outta of the relationship.

And that is often when the guy phones our office for an appointment and says, "My wife says she's leaving. I knew she wasn't thrilled, but I had no idea it was as awful as this, and I want to do something. I love her and I want her, and I'll do anything to change. Help me. I'm desperate to save this marriage."

And it's too late. She undoubtedly is done.

All that *niceness* builds up resentment and pain and distance. *Niceness*—suppressing good old honest anger that could, if expressed, clear up the little nigglings inevitable in all relationships. In the end, all that niceness contributes to the demise of the relationship.

For many women it seems marginally crazy to actively express anger as a way of building relationship and enhancing connection. The thought of making your spouse profoundly uncomfortable appears absurd. Can it actually be a good idea to boldly speak about what's not working for you? For many women, actively teaching your husband how to be a husband to you, with your dreams and plans, your styles and quirks, seems counterintuitive to being a good wife.

But it's not.

We often see kindness and niceness as interchangeable, but they aren't. Sometimes the behaviors expressed out of being "nice" and "kind" appear similar. However, kindness and niceness are fundamentally different qualities.

***

Let me explain the difference:

Niceness is being pleasant and agreeable in a way for it to be easy for others to be around and hear what you are saying. It's about being socially or conventionally correct.

Kindness is about being tender and considerate and helpful. It shows mercy and compassion. There is a courage to authentic kindness.

So, kindness and niceness at first can seem very similar—and in fact, have overlap. But the focus is very different.

Being **nice** is self-focused. What do I need to do so others will perceive me well; so I will fit in and be liked? What would society or this community expect of me as a spouse, and what "should" I do to deliver? It is shame based. It is trying to act in a way to be loved and accepted: What can I do to be seen as good enough? Niceness has its roots in fear. Niceness says: "What thing can I do so that people will judge me positively?"

Being **kind** is other focused. It's about compassion and empathy for the person in front of you. Kindness cares enough to do what is necessary to relieve suffering without regard for what others will think. It's based in confidence, secure in oneself and one's own identity to do exactly what needs to be done. Kindness has its roots in love. In marriage, kindness says, "What is the next right thing to do that will make my partner and our marriage stronger? How can I truly and bravely say what needs to be said?"

Kindness sits down and listens to your spouse carefully, even when it's heavy and painful.

Niceness quickly says, "It'll be fine. We don't have to talk about it."

Kindness holds space for the easy and the hard stuff of a relationship.

Nice expects your partner to gloss over the ugly parts.

Kindness risks saying, "If you're asking me for my opinion, I don't like the idea."

Nice wishes you well without authenticity.

Kindness says, "I care enough about our marriage to give you information that will be inconvenient for you to hear. You may respond in a way that is defensive or challenging, and I won't let that stop me."

Nice says, "I don't want to handle you getting upset, so I'll just stay silent over this piece that doesn't work".

Kindness says, "I choose to invest in our relationship by having a difficult conversation with you because we are worth it."

Nice says, "Forget about it. Not that big of a deal."

Kindness says, "I bring up a difficult topic about how something isn't working for me in our marriage. I don't want to set you up to hurt me when you don't realize what bothers me. It's not fair to be angry and resentful about your behavior when I haven't been respectful enough to let you be aware."

Nice says, "I'm gonna grit my teeth and pretend you don't irritate me because it's too awkward to let you know something really bugs me."

Niceness involves pleasantness at all times. Inherent in niceness is a level of dishonesty. It's often not well received, because it doesn't have depth. How many of you have had a conversation with your spouse where you have smiled through gritted teeth? Where you went through the motions of getting along, all the while feeling a hypocrite?

I suspect you have had occasion to smell niceness a mile away from your partner. When you could feel it, you probably didn't trust it.

Kindness feels honest. Kindness calls deep on courage. It's brave to be truly kind. It means being authentic and deeply loving. Kind requires taking risks and investing deeply in relationships, knowing it will become uncomfortable sometimes.

***

One of the most challenging tasks for me as a therapist who works with couples is to get people to stop being so nice to each other. They have *niced the life* right out of their marriage. It's a shell of politeness but there's little engagement, no depth, and little trust. There's not a lot of difficult discussion happening—because that wouldn't be nice, right? And eventually, there's almost no conversation.

A big part of my job with these couples is to get them to realize that it is kind and caring to get messy. I work to draw on their courage to raise issues of workload or finances, around sex, or whatever is concerning and upsetting. When couples start authentically connecting over the real stuff of life—they get terrified about having the conversations.

However, when a couple chooses kind over nice, it is really the first day of their real marriage. Scary but real. Like the mythical velveteen rabbit who became real when he had bare spots in the fabric and a missing ear, a real relationship will have discussions that are raw and messy.

There may be a conversation that sounds suspiciously like an argument. It will be messy. And it may take more than one conversation to figure out how to really hear each other. You may have to read a book or talk to a therapist as external resources to navigate through the muddy waters of honest conflict.

Kind conversations require courage that nice conversations do not.

But your marriage will emerge strong.

Expressing clearly and effectively what isn't working is a gift you give your spouse. Because when it isn't working for you, it isn't working for anybody.

When it works for you and your spouse both—then it is working for everybody.

Let this book have you think through how to talk to your spouse about your discomfort in your marriage.

Some chapters won't apply to your circumstance…no need to read those. Grab ideas of how to communicate. Remember phrases that say what you feel in ways you've never been able to articulate. Highlight portions that speak your heart, your pain, your dreams. Use this book in whatever way is helpful for you to have a better relationship.

This book isn't therapy, nor is it intended to replace therapy. It is a chance to be real with yourselves and each other about the *state of your union*. Once you become honest with yourselves and each other, then together you can figure out a plan.

I believe in couple therapy. Of course I do. I do couple therapy with couples and I see it work. I see couples get stronger, figure things out, reconnect with each other, find their first love. As much as it might be expensive; as challenging and vulnerable as it might be, therapy may actually be the best option for you.

Couple therapy isn't cheap, but it is priceless!

Find a path that works for the two of you, with your own quirks and interests and style. But make sure it works for both of you. Keep at it, try different things until something works.

Your marriage is worth the hassle of figuring out the difference between kind and nice.

.

2 IF IT AIN'T WORKIN' FOR BOTH OF YOU, IT AIN'T WORKIN'

Dear Wives-who-are-lonely,

This is a horrifying statistic: Women initiate 69 percent of divorces.[i]

Over 2/3's of divorces occur because the wives say, "Enough".

I want husbands to have a chance to learn that it isn't working before it's too late. As a marriage therapist, I've met few husbands who don't care about their wives, and intentionally ignore their relationship. So many husbands are gob smacked when their wives tell them they are done.

Wives—you didn't get married expecting it to end. I appreciate you had dreams and hopes about the future.

And somewhere, things went sideways.

You're likely tired and frustrated. And I'm sorry that it seems exhausting and demoralizing to be living the life you are in.

If you're the typical wife, you do an hour more of housework per day than your husband,[ii] You spend double the time caring for others than he does. It's difficult to do so much of the heavy lifting around the house.

First, being responsible for so much is just plain hard. Maybe you also work full time. But even more, the difference in workloads is just plain unjust. It's hard not to be resentful when he's tired and relaxing in front of the TV, and you're tired and making lunches for the next day.

I recognize you are doing the best you can…and if you're like most women, you've been taught that a good woman doesn't complain, she does what it takes to make everything work.

When he needs extra time at work, you pick up the slack. When he gets away with the guys and tells you he needs a break, you take on single parenting duties without missing a beat. When the playoffs are on, you work to fill the house with snacks for him and his friends. You work hard to be supportive of him. As Dr. Gottman would say, you accept influence from your husband naturally. [iii]

When you have a business trip, you leave notes about what everybody needs to do and when.

If you are out to a book club for the evening, you paste on a frozen grin when your mother says, "Isn't it nice he babysits so you can go out?" Because you know, you raise the children, and he babysits. (NOT!!) It's not like she would say she doesn't support you, or want you to have your own time—she isn't even aware of her language.

And you recognize that given the pace of the family, it makes little sense to apply for a promotion at work. (Even though neither of you would think to have him slow his progress up the ladder at his employment.)

Wife-who-feels-ignored, can I tell you something that is honest, but perhaps hard for you to believe?

The husband in your life doesn't get it. He genuinely doesn't.

If you ask him, he will probably say he does half-the-work-of-the-household-*ish*. He doesn't appreciate how much more you do that he isn't even aware. He also sees you generally cheerful and mostly cooperative as you go about doing so much—which is true, because you like making a home for your family. You wouldn't dream of guilting your kids or your mother for what you do for them, right?

***

I think the many husbands of this world don't recognize that their marriages are slowing diminishing. (And there are some wives that don't get it either.)

You are disappearing from your marriage slowly, drop by drop, and your husband doesn't even notice.

You may have just found your eyes suddenly begin to leak. You teared up now because you felt, at last, understood. This marriage isn't life-giving like you dreamed it would be—as your husband believes it still is.

In my experience as a therapist, women are often much unhappier in the marriage than the husband realizes. Often she comes to therapy alone, desperate to change something. Her husband will not come to therapy for any number of excuses which all boil down to one reason: he doesn't want to come to therapy.

To be fair, therapy involves talking about feelings, something men are raised to believe is not something they are good at. And actually, some men really aren't good at it. How many of us can do anything well when we have never done it before?

If men in his life did not model it for him or showed him how to talk about emotion, how is he supposed to know? Men are taught in our culture that says people who go to therapy to talk about feelings are wusses or sissies.

And what are men called who go to therapy because their wives ask them to? Well, there are several names for those sorts of men. None of them positive.

You're dying inside as you live in a marriage that looks good from the outside: you're paying down the mortgage, going on a vacation with the kids, putting money into RRSP's and maybe going out for dinner on Friday night. It all looks pretty good.

Except it ain't workin' for you—and hasn't for a long time.

I have had clients who were wives that were wonderful women willing and ready to over-function as a sign of their love for the first several years of their marriage. Young brides can be cheerfully dismissive how he goes off with the boys, buys big-ticket items for his own leisure with joint funds, and forgets to put his dishes away etc. etc. Most wives can live in the mundane routine of a marriage while being taken for granted for a decade or so. But when the kids come along, and the amount of work goes up exponentially, his disregard for her disproportionate efforts stops being cute and gets annoying. But he's used to under-functioning and doesn't understand how serious it is.

Dear-wives-who-are-being-ignored, this isn't nearly all about housework either, is it? This is about the man who promised to support you and be your engaged partner in your life, now:

- tunes you out while he plays video games
- plans his weekend and then has you plan around his plans
- is unaware of how tired you are
- does not check in with you about your day's experiences, or what you would choose as the

family's next big project to save for, or maybe just
about doesn't check in with you at all

And, wives-who-are-lonely, some of you are so discouraged, that
you are putting in time until the kids are older, or are already
planning your exit—and he doesn't know it.

I get it.

Our culture says nice women work hard and don't complain.

No one wants to be a "witch with a b". Women are used to being
the one responsible for resolving the conflict and maintaining the
wellbeing of the relationship.

So, women keep the peace in a relationship that isn't working well
for them by:

- speaking up—but not too loudly
- stating her concerns—but so gently the severity of
  the concerns is lost
- avoid and put off stating how much this hurts
  because you don't want to hurt his feelings
- deciding that the hassle of telling him this isn't
  working for you isn't worth it because you
  know he will minimize, joke around, blow you off,
  or start a fight that won't end until you give in and
  go quiet, and smile nicely

…and meanwhile, the marriage is rotting silently from the inside
out.

It is unfortunate he doesn't notice on his own. It is
also unfortunate you protect him from the knowing his marriage is
heading towards its demise. He's taught you he won't hear and
won't respond, and so it's easier not to try. He can detect the
wiggle room to fool himself that it is "just your time of the
month", or the baby has kept you up, or…

16

I've met men like your husbands, and they will be completely bamboozled when you leave. Because they are clueless about how difficult it is for you.

***

Can I ask you a favor, wife-who-is-lonely?

Can you make it crystal clear to him that this isn't working and that he needs to step up?

Do it in a way he **can't** miss it. Let him know you aren't just complaining about the glass on the counter, or about one night with the guys, or about how he didn't empty the dishwasher yesterday.

Let him realize this is a serious situation where you yearn to be known and understood by the guy who once had you feel you were the most important person in the world. Tell him that there is a deep concern about the long-term fundamental wellbeing of this marriage. Share with him that he is missing out on meaningful engagement with you as his wife.

This isn't whining.

You aren't griping.

You are looking him in the eye and respecting him enough to raise an important issue before it is too late.

Make it different from all the other conversations you've ever had about your marriage. Identify a way to have him feel the gravity. Maybe you'll have to do something drastic in a creative, significant, even very serious way that creates a shift he can't ignore. Let him know you're tired and missing him, and longing for him to be in tune with you—and the consequences of not doing relationship repair will be dire. That at some point, you may leave the marriage formally because for you, the marriage will actually have been dead for some time.

This won't be mean or bitchy.

***

To let him know this marriage is not working for you is the ultimate act of kindness from you to him.

Because he needs to appreciate if this marriage isn't working for one of you, it isn't working for either of you.

Even if it feels to him like the marriage is good for him as is, if it isn't sustainable and he gets left alone, that will suck for him. Big time.

Can I ask you another favor?

When you let him understand, with absolute clarity and huge vulnerability and great courage, would you also give him the benefit of the doubt?

Don't label him a jerk. Don't call him names. Be respectful and remind him of how he matters enough to you to risk being open with him.

Remind him of your vows, your dreams and hopes together. Challenge him to align his behavior with his core values of love for family and for you. It's quite possible he really loves you, and he is not aware of how much he takes you for granted.

His behavior is not good, but if you attack his character rather than his behavior, he doesn't have a lot of room to respond positively. You want him to leave the conversation knowing you believe he can do better, because he is better than that.

***

He might be really pissed.

I mean, really, *really* pissed.

No guy likes to know the person who matters most to him finds him falling short. It is so much easier to be pissed than crushed, devastated, or deeply regretful, especially for men. Give him a day or two to wrap his head around it. Give him time to calm down and then talk about it.

But understand many husbands will hope that situation will "blow over" in a few days.

Don't let it blow over.

Calmly and assertively let him know no action is experienced as continued disengagement, and you are really pulling for him to invest in the relationship. Many will find counseling a great option. A therapist will help your husband understand his behaviour. We don't believe in blaming people; we stand for changing patterns to be constructive.

Some of you might do a marriage enrichment weekend, engage in an online course. Take a survey. You can find lots of great resources online.

Others of you might just benefit from reading books, Friends of mine each purchased the same popular book about vital marriages, and have formed a mini-book club.

Just the two of them.

They highlight the parts that seem relevant and compare what each wrote. They write in the margins about how what they are reading applies to them. And then they sit down together to go through the book, page by page, reading it out loud to each other, and stopping as often as needed, to really determine how to relate it to their own marriage.

He won't go to therapy?

Watch movies! There is research that says when couples that watch a movie together from a designated list of movies and then discuss them afterwards, they can have substantial improvements in their relationships,[iv] (Remember though, the value of this occurs when there is quality discussion after the movie.)

Do *something*.

And then try something else if it doesn't work for both of you.

Change the trajectory of your marriage. Don't let him silently coerce you to remain in a marriage you are aware is slowly dying. Be clear with him that continuing with his benign disengagement is destructive and make it hard for him to fool himself otherwise.

Here's to hoping you find the strength to pull off what is truly the most challenging and important conversation of your life!

3 BEFORE IT IS TOO LATE

I was talking recently to some of my colleagues about couples' therapy.

One topic that came up was the reluctance of one partner to pick up on the other spouse's pain...and do something about it.

Sometimes, when couples come to therapy, it is very apparent one partner has very much desired to come, and the other is attending very reluctantly. It's then a therapist asks the couples which one is the "draggee" in therapy, and one the "dragger".

A therapist mentioned the painful scenario of having a couple come into therapy after one spouse has said:

Enough. I'm done:

- Enough of the distance,
- Enough of trying to make the partner understand the loneliness.
- Enough of pleading, trying to make something happen.
- Enough of saying, "We need to talk to somebody. We need to figure this out."

- Enough of trying to have their spouse learn this isn't just some disgruntlement about the schedule or the chores. This isn't some bickering or complaining that will pass.
- Enough of not being heard.
- Enough of not being seen and valued

The exhausted, burned out spouse says:

"Enough. I'm not doing this anymore. I'm done."

And means it.

***

Suddenly the spouse hears the pain, and understands the seriousness of the marital crisis. The one trying for so long has started packing. The years of effort are over.

The spouse now *gets it*. **Big time.**

The spouse kicks into high gear (because all along s/he really wanted to be married, but you know how complacency can set in). In horror and shock, the spouse begins to plead for the marriage.

***

Sincerely, dedicatedly, and earnestly, the spouse:

- Books the counseling appointment
- Tries to start conversations, writes long letters of love and commitment, texts love and commitment multiple times per day
- Now comes home from work on time
- Fixes the things that have been on the "to do list" for months
- Actively takes part in childcare
- Shows up at the kids' games

...in short, doing all the things that have been complained about for eons.

The imminence of divorce propels action in frenetic ways.

Only it's too late.

When "enough" was announced, it was too late.

The last chances had already been offered and re-offered, and had already been pulled off the table.

When one therapist said this to the rest of us, there were sad smiles of knowing all around the room. We've all seen these couples and its painful.

The sad part is when these couples show up for therapy, the draggee has become the dragger, and now, the dragger has become the draggee.

The formerly-begging-and-pleading spouse is done with the marriage. They come to therapy only to have the therapist's help to explain that there is no more opportunity to work on this.

Therapists generally only see these couples once, because there is nothing to do, nothing to work on. There is no intention on the part of the one who is done to re-engage. She will say she's tried over and over for years and is done trying.

The spouse that hadn't been accessible and responsive really is sincere about wanting to make the marriage work (and has wanted to be married all along). And as motivated as they now might be, there is no space to make the marriage work—because **there is no marriage** anymore.

The marriage disintegrated in front of their eyes, but they didn't see it—because their eyes were glued to the video game, the football game, the beer in front of them, or the project at work.

Statistically, frankly, this spouse is most often (though not nearly always) male.

The long pattern of distancing isn't about being a jerk. It's *about the challenge of being intimate with someone in a culture that ridicules vulnerability and makes it difficult.* It's about pulling away from someone who makes you feel like you are never enough and can never measure up.

It's turning away from something you feel lousy at, to move towards an area where you have competence—like your job or the hockey team, or an area of mindless numbing like video games or alcohol.

So often, these men value and love their wives, and want a good marriage, but don't know how, and they pull away from the uncomfortable feelings...

...and don't realize that this results in pulling away from your life's love in ways that seem intolerable to her.

***

This book is designed to start an important conversation.

This book is for her—to develop language and courage to speak up; to have difficult conversations that seem easier to not have on any given day—except then they might never occur. This book is for you to contemplate if the high price of making change is actually lower than the high price of staying silent in a relationship where the drift creates an ever widening distance.

This book is for him—to show him sections that stand out to you. Highlight bits you want him to see. This book can be a powerful symbol to him that change is required: a slowing of schedules, an increased engagement, a step up to take part more in the tasks of the household. This book is to help him hear how desperate you are to connect with him in a meaningfully.

This book dares you to figure out how to make this work for both of you...before it's too late.

.

4 *TOO MUCH* CAN SQUASH A MARRIAGE

Boiling water for tea is a great thing unless it's *too much*.

When it's too much, it's just not a good thing. Even though boiling water for tea is a fairly benign activity.

Let me explain.

At our clinic, we don't use the harsh overhead fluorescent lights in the counseling rooms. My thinking is that uncovering and exposing parts of oneself is hard enough without seeming like you are under glaring floodlights. So the overhead lights are off, and there is much more muted and soft lighting from several floor and desk lamps about each of the counseling offices.

In the cooler months, our offices hold the chill. Being a corner office, we have two outside walls, and the heating from the building's central heating system doesn't warm it up enough. So we have space heaters in each office and the main area. People are feeling "on edge" often when they come to see us—so trying to warm up the environment and increase the cozy factor is important. (Which all sounds so altruistic. To be frank, it's hard for me to facilitate good therapy with a client when my teeth are chattering and my fingers are cold, so it works for me, too)

Melanie, our office manager, likes to work under the fluorescents, so they are on in the main office area where she is. However, she also has a desk lamp on her desk. Our fabulous interior designer, Robyn, says a person is 30 percent more productive with a desk lamp. I'm all over research...thus the lamp. The "30 percent productivity increase" has become something of quirky office lore.

Our administration space is, ahem, efficient in its use of space (which is another way of saying a terribly cramped). So, in a piece of furniture that originally built as an armoire contains our "kitchen". We use the lower drawers for office supplies, and the large open space that would normally hold a television now is the "kitchen". It holds a little fridge, our microwave and kettle.

So, with the lamps on in the counseling room, on Melanie's desk, the fridge going, and starting in the fall, the space heaters, when we plug in the kettle to make tea—all at once, it goes dark and silent.

The breaker pops. We are drawing too much power on a circuit.

And Melanie makes a dash to the breaker panel to bring the lights back on in the therapy session next door.

By Christmas, Melanie will have retrained us. Before we put the kettle on, we unplug the heater and announce to her we will be decreasing her efficiency (temporarily) by 30 percent.

The kettle itself is not the obstacle. The heaters' seasonal use is not the issue. The lamps aren't the problem.

The complication is having too many of them drawing power all at once from a system that has finite levels of capability. Using all the devices at once exceeds that capacity.

***

Exhaustion has become something of a status symbol in our culture. When people say, "How are you?", one of the common

27

(and unfortunately, respected) answers is "Really busy" or "Really tired" or "Very stressed".

How is it we, as a way of life, esteem those who are maxed out?

Somewhere along the way, people determine their value on their level of productivity. With our very value on the line, folks exhaust themselves to prove how valuable they are, maybe even indispensable.

When we base a person's value on their productivity, exhaustion is the logical, even inevitable, outcome. When we hinge a parent's worth as a parent on how many activities that their children are involved in, the children and parents are overbooked and overloaded. It is an unreasonable expectation for a parent to watch every game and sit through each lesson—when the kids are overscheduled themselves.

There is a cost to relationships when either or both partners are exhausted. Some circuit breakers somewhere in the relationship break at some point because *too much* is: **Just. Too. Much.**

***

I had a conversation with a colleague recently who wryly commented that breaking her arm had been the best thing that happened to her marriage this summer.

She couldn't golf with her buddies, nobody asked her to play as a sub for the baseball team, she couldn't take on new projects in the yard, and so on. Because of her injury, by necessity, she had to just *be*.

She was less exhausted because she didn't/couldn't have as much on her "to do" list. With the additional time and the extra "gas in her tank", she and her husband had a renaissance of sorts in their relationship. They spent time walking in the neighborhood, got hooked on a series on Netflix that they would watch together (and dissect after). They cooked together and ate together more than they had in ages.

And she loved it.

***

Years ago, my financial planner encouraged me to purchase "catastrophic illness insurance" so that if I contracted any one of a list of serious medical illnesses, I would be immediately qualify for a large cash payment. I could use the extra cash towards unexpected medical expenses. However, he said many people had life-changing mind-set changes. They might now want to take a trip with their families, or cut back on how hard they were working. He noted that in the face of catastrophic illness, there was often a shift in priorities towards relationships and creating memories. This insurance accommodates for these shifts by allowing a person to pull back from their financial obligations to pursue their newly realigned values.

This thought horrified me then and still does now.

One of my most heartfelt prayers for my life is that I would not need a "wake up call" like a catastrophic illness to be fully alive to the relationships significant to me. I don't want a diagnosis to prompt me to adjust my schedule to something that works.

I want to make choices to live out what I know to be meaningful now while I'm healthy.

***

The little important things can so easily get lost amid the busy-ness: the little touch of romance with lighting a candle for the meal, cutting a blossom and bringing it inside to put in a vase, rubbing sore feet at the end of the day, or drawing a hot bath for a spouse.

Those little expressions of kindness and care take time and energy, which rarely exists in our maxed-out culture.

Checking Facebook (and YouTube, and Twitter, and email and a blog and the news highlights and...), taking on another project at work, accepting the promotion, figuring out how to move to a bigger house, enrolling the kids in one more sport, agreeing to one additional committee...all of these can put us into situations where we max out the circuit and something has gotta give.

None of these are bad, but the stress on the system is HUGE.

For some couples I have seen for marital counseling, the therapy session serves as the one and only time in the week where they can be 100 percent focused on each other. Where a couple listens deeply, and the only opportunity to feel heard (and valued and appreciated) by their partner. The rest of the week is too much of a scramble. There is no other time possible to simply sit quietly with each other and focus on themselves as a couple.

I think sometimes folks put investing in their marriage "on hold" when things get busy, and promise themselves that they will tend to it, when they can, later.

If later ever comes.

When the circuit is too full, even full of good stuff, the breaker can turn it all off.

It's heartbreaking to watch a couple come in with their marriage in a serious crisis because there have been far too many draws of energy.

A marriage cannot survive unlimited additions of tasks, interests, distractions and stressors. Any relationship will collapse under the onslaught of prolonged over-scheduling.

The breaker will pop.

How much power are you drawing off? I have witnessed folks who have spent years driving their children around to many lessons and practices, had grueling work schedules to generate enough income for a certain standard of living. They drive themselves to exhaustion. Folks run themselves into the ground, "for the sake of the family".

Your family wants your husband and you even more than they want a raise. You want your husband's time and energy and investment more than you want a new car or an expensive vacation, right? Your children may complain if they can't get the newest gaming system. However, that pain pales compared to not having two parents engaged with them, playing in the yard or cheering from the bleachers.

Consider calling your husband over to read this. Or your wife. Perhaps the two of you have a distance between you because one or both of you have such full plates that your marriage isn't being nurtured.

A neglected relationship deteriorates.

Have a discussion about how to recalibrate your energies and decide what to take out of your life before life decides for you.

Know too much of a good thing is too much. You could lose the **important** as you get distracted by the **urgent**.

5 DISENGAGEMENT…THE SILENT, SLIPPERY BETRAYAL

Have you even thought of disengagement as betrayal?

We usually think of betrayal in terms of infidelity—affairs. When a spouse is unfaithful in engaging in a sexual relationship with another—that's clearly betrayal. Or when a partner has an intimate emotional relationship, even if it doesn't culminate with sex in the relationship—most would also see this as betrayal.

Other common betrayals which hit the must-go-see-therapist-in-crisis threshold?

- significant financial mismanagement or secret spending resulting in the discovery of a scary pile of debt
- drug use or obsessive porn viewing or gambling discovery. The disclosure of a secret; the discovery of engagement in an undesirable activity; or the surprise of a hidden credit card statement

It is absolutely necessary to deal with the shock and horror that has a couple reeling after a cataclysmic betrayal. Facing the other way and continuing on like it didn't happen is rather like building on sand. It might look normal on the outside, but inside each partner is insecurity, fear, sadness and mistrust. Underneath what looks fine lies a shaky foundation.

A good deal of the time, however, a spouse might gradually discover a silent, more insidious betrayal. A betrayal begun a long time before one of those obvious betrayals, slowly eroding the underlying base of the relationship, priming it for disaster.

Brene Brown writes about disengagement in her best-selling book, Daring Greatly:

> In fact, this betrayal usually happens long before the other ones. I'm talking about the betrayal of disengagement. Of not caring. Of letting the connection go. Of not being willing to devote time and effort to the relationship. The word betrayal evokes experiences of cheating, lying, breaking a confidence, failing to defend us to someone else who's gossiping about us, and not choosing us over other people. These behaviors are certainly betrayals, but they're not the only form of betrayal. If I had to choose the form of betrayal that emerged most frequently from my research and that was the most dangerous in terms of corroding the trust connection, I would say disengagement.[v]

Let me be clear, people: this ain't no frivolous line I found in some obscure book.

This is something we see regularly at our counseling office. Often when couples show up with a marriage in shambles, disengagement has had an enormous, though largely hidden, effect on the marriage.

Disengagement is sneaky.

Disengagement is hard to name. It's hard to talk about. And harder to actually figure out what to do about it.

***

The betrayal of disengagement is:

- Often written off as a partner "making a mountain out of a molehill".
- Pawned off as "well, boys will be boys", giving a legitimacy to the practice of ignoring the primary relationship in a husband's life. He spends night after night watching hockey with the guys, a beer in his hand.
- Explained/rationalized as necessary e.g. "I have to put all these hours in at the business or it will fail." How do you argue against a line like that?
- Minimized as insignificant: "C'mon, it's only hanging out in the workshop getting little things done…it's my alone time. It's not like I'm having an affair with a woman. What's the big deal? Don't you want me to enjoy my life?"

When a partner feels disengagement and raises the concern:

- She is called out as being whiny or a drama queen
- She dares not express the loneliness because you know what's coming…She will be labelled as a needy or worse yet, high maintenance. Why would any woman want to raise the issue of a partner's disengagement if that will happen?
- She simply doesn't have the opportunity to discuss the concern because some level of engagement would be required to even start the conversation…and between the incredible number of hours at work, and the children: They. Never. Connect.

Brené Brown also says:

When the people we love or with whom we have a deep connection stop caring, stop paying attention, stop investing and fighting for the relationship, trust begins to slip away and hurt starts seeping in. Disengagement triggers shame and our greatest fears - the fears of being abandoned, unworthy, and unlovable. What can make this covert betrayal so much more dangerous than something like a lie or an affair is that we can't point to the source of our pain - there's no event, no obvious evidence of brokenness. It can feel crazy-making.[vi]

"There's no event, no obvious evidence of brokenness. It can feel crazy making." Does that feel like truth inside of you when you read it?

***

The toll of disengagement is high.

Very high.

It takes a toll on the relationship. It creates a vulnerability in the relationship as broad as a barn door for the marriage to become like the walking dead. It looks like it's all there, but it is so not.

The cost of disengagement is a hollow marriage, that limps along with a focus on the children, with little more in common than a mailing address. Both partners are disengaged, and don't invest in the relationship to change it.

Sometimes, in desperation, the partner that has experienced the disengagement resorts to behaviour out of line with his/her values to cope with the pain of the fears and shame. An affair. Alcohol. Excessive shopping. We all know what happens in these situations.

And it ain't pretty. Trust me.

I don't know of anyone who has entered a marriage thinking,

- "When it gets hard or busy or risky, I'm going to step back without acknowledging it," or
- "When I am not heard, I'll give up trying," or
- "If my spouse doesn't hear me when I express a concern, I'll just pull away and put my interests elsewhere."

Nobody does that.

Not intentionally, anyway.

***

Inviting a spouse to authentic engagement is risky, daring, courageous work:

It means raising a stink over something that is covert, hidden and insidious. Your partner probably won't understand. Your spouse may be frustrated with you seemingly making something out of nothing. A disengaged partner who rarely drifts away it intentionally or maliciously. The drift happens without them noticing.

It's hard to raise an issue when it feels like your concern could be brushed off. That often feels like you've been brushed off...and nobody likes that.

***

You may want to show your partner this chapter...to demonstrate to your partner you are not crazy, you are not making this up, that the distance between the two of you has a name: *disengagement*. And your partner can learn that with disengagement, there is pain. Always. For both.

It might mean calling in a therapist to help you say to your partner, "I am intolerably lonely. And this situation is not sustainable," with the therapist helping you to be heard. The experience of disengagement then becomes a conversation with a counselor, and that gives you the space to go at it differently. You can figure out how to work on it.

Re-engaging may prevent rash, inappropriate and highly expensive behaviour that will create social, relational, family, psychological costs for years to come. Extramarital affairs are sometimes a logical outcome of disengagement. I'm not legitimizing them as an inevitable result. I'm describing reality.

Be honest with yourself. And then with your spouse about disengagement.

**And spouse of the person reading this book? If your partner has called you over to look at this page, please know it is serious. Engage in a curious, compassionate conversation that explores why she wanted you to read it. Please? Know that being shown this chapter is a tentative, brave and maybe desperate signal to wake up and pay attention. Being shown this chapter, quite simply, is a gift I'm inviting you to accept. A hard gift (painful, but given out of care and desire to make things better)

6 IT'S IMPORTANT TO HURT HIS FEELINGS

It's important to hurt his feelings.

Hers too, for that matter.

***

Jim, my husband, is good for me. He is so good at marriage.

Jim teaches me so much about what it feels like to be in a good relationship, it sometimes takes my breath away.

One thing Jim does is invite me to tell him when, from my perspective, something isn't working. Even if it will be hard for him to receive.

That doesn't sit easily with me. I don't relish the thought of saying something to him that will be hurtful or be uncomfortable for him.

So, although it often feels like I'm opening Pandora's box, and I don't know how it will go, I let him know when I'm not feeling right about something he is doing, because that's what he asks.

We were having a conversation the other day about some plans we were making, and he said, "You're quiet...what are you thinking?"

My immediate response?

"Nothing." I muttered.

Which wasn't true.

But it was my first impulse. A lot of us say, "Nothing" as a stock answer. "Nothing," is easier than, "Well, the something I want to say is a something you're not gonna like".

Maybe you do that too?

***

But then I remember: that's not how Jim and I roll. That's not what he asks for me.

So I take a deep breath, and wade into saying something that is honest, but not easy.

It isn't easy because: I recognize it will probably hurt his feelings.

I jump into the deep end. I identified how this conversation felt like past patterns. I felt the conversation was headed in a direction that felt familiar and typically unsuccessful, so I fell silent. I let him know that I felt this conversation was headed towards futility. I'll spare you the details, but I essentially accused Jim of a negative behaviour.

His answer shocked me. After a moment of silence, he said: "Thank you for telling me. I'm really glad you said something."

That's how he started: "Thank you".

Gratitude.

It's not the first time, in fact, it's his usual response when I say something that might feel hurtful to him.

Crazy wonderful!

It speaks to Jim's character that his first response is gratitude when I dare tell him something hard. It also makes it easier for me to talk to him the next time.

I could sense how it was a deliberate decision for him to say thank you. I'm not sure it is the instinct of most of us to first invite criticism and then be grateful for it.

It wasn't easy for him to hear, but it was helpful in moving our conversation forward. Because the dialogue that followed was powerful. It impacted the way we talk about planning, not just in this conversation, but all future conversations. A path for us to pursue "together" better.

He acknowledged my hesitation and fears. Jim owned who he is, and he owned what he has done in the past. He heard my perspective. He let me experience he had heard it by re-telling me what he had heard me say, leaving no doubt. Only then, did he gave me his thoughts. His perspective was important and his gracious response gave me the grace to hear it.

We had a great conversation about how we plan, and how we can better plan so it works for both of us.

I think we're a stronger couple for it.

***

Jim also knows I'm human.

I possess tender spots that predate him. They don't always make sense because I've had a lifetime of experiences unique to me that have shaped me. Sometimes I get hurt when others wouldn't. I have quirks and preferences unique to me—and he isn't aware about these unless I tell him. He gets that.

Jim invites me to be me, and that means he invites me to let him know when something he does is uncomfortable for me.

I think it is incredible—he has shaped our conversation so my "complaints" about what he does are hurdles we have to figure out together, rather than something he becomes defensive about.

***

My initial silence was my default response—our cultural climate has trained so many of us:

"If you can't say something nice, say nothing at all."

And so when something isn't working, no one knows. No one can do anything about it.

Nothing happens.

And whatever isn't working well between the two in the relationship stays not working.

***

It's probably strange to hear a therapist tell you how important it is to hurt another person's feelings.

It's strange for me to write it.

To be frank, one reason us therapists have as many clients as we do is in the effort to avoid hurting another person's feelings, many important conversations never happen.

When important conversations remain unspoken, then something that isn't working stays not working.

If it merely stayed not working, that would be problem enough.

Picture that unspoken conversation as a snowball rolling down a hill, gathering momentum with every moment of silence. The longer that conversation remains unspoken, the more the unspoken conversation affects the relationship.

Topics such as the way you and he spend money, sex happens (or doesn't happen) or things get done (or don't get done) around the house builds and builds.

By not processing and working through the problem, it gains in size and speed. As time marches on, the problems snowball.

And, over the course of a couple decades, *avoiding the conversation so you don't hurt his/her feelings* can destroy the relationship.

***

I think it's helpful to hurt a person's feelings.

Emotions are information for us—our feelings help us learn important things at a deep level. Hurt feelings don't kill people. (Even though we sometimes feel and act like they do). When people are hurting, it gives them something to be curious about; something they can work with to move forward in ways that make them better, stronger, more compassionate people.

Hurt feelings are a normal response by a normal person to what is happening in the world.

Those hurt feelings are a tremendous motivation to change future behaviour in ways that enhance the relationship and make the world a better place.

***

Jim and I have a commitment: *to raise something that doesn't feel right as soon as possible.*

We decided early on we didn't want the other one saving us from a hard, hurtful conversation if it could mean the unspoken conversation might create relationship rot.

Our commitment is to have conversations that might hurt the other person's feelings. To not have those conversations is to hurt both of us much more in the big picture.

To be clear, we don't have the conversations *with the agenda to hurt* the other's feelings. That's not the intention, just a by-product we will accept.

We work to reduce/minimize or even eliminate the pain by how we craft the conversation.

A few of our strategies to reduce the pain of the other, or be compassionate towards it when it happens:

- We allow ourselves to experience the discomfort and work through it. Sometimes, Jim will tell me he has thought about how to word a conversation for several days before he raises the issue. I'm glad, even if he takes time, he finds a way, eventually.
- We work to approach it as a team. If I'm driving him nuts, he knows this is something we have to figure out together. He trusts I don't get up in the morning intending to make his life miserable. None of us do. However, isn't it interesting how sometimes, we talk to our partner as if they are out to make our lives miserable?
- We stay civil. Kind and gentle. The style with which you bring something up speaks to your spirit. People respond to the spirit of the conversation more than the words. Jim is never nasty. I can hear his complaint about how I did something so much easier when he has a soft start up to the conversation.

43

- The conversation is just that—a conversation. When one of us raises a concern, we find out where the other person was coming from. Often that allows for both of us to hear where the other person was coming from; why it made sense at some level for things to happen the way they did. Discovering new details about each other and ourselves is an important part of the process to get to a richer new place in our relationship.
- We remind ourselves, sometimes in the middle of a conversation, that talking about this stuff is hard. We also remind ourselves that not talking about this stuff, is ultimately, harder. *Yes, seriously, we do.*

These conversations happen only occasionally. In between these conversations there is lots of laughter. We have fun times. Lot of affirmations of love and appreciation. We remind each other that we see each other as a fabulous partners. We remind each other we deliberately chose each other. We built our relationship to handle hard conversations that might be hurtful.

***

Jim and I do not have a perfect relationship.

Far from it. The above list is something we work towards...and fail at. And when we do, one of us can get hurt—and then we work to resolve it—using the list as outlined above.

Rinse and repeat.

We're human, just like anybody else. But one strength of our relationship is the ability we have given each other to bring up when something isn't working.

We are playing the long game which means working out the

wrinkles as they arise so they don't hijack the relationship.

***

Jim says something occasionally that is helpful to hear:

> "I'm glad you're not perfect. Because I'm not perfect. And if you were perfect, you wouldn't have married me."

When he says that, it helps me to not feel as wounded when he brings something up. He doesn't expect, or even want me to not make mistakes. It makes it so much easier for me to say, "Thank you for telling me that" when he raises an issue with something I've done.

I love that he deliberately creates room for me to make mistakes, mess up, apologize and move on.

Have I mentioned that he's good for me?

Can you invite your spouse to a conversation where you might leave wounded? Would you give your partner the gift of being able to hold your own pain if it would be good for the relationship in the long run?

7 WORK ON THE CONNECTION NOT THE COMMUNICATION

"We all fear facing life alone and we all long for loving connection – a hand to hold that changes our world to a safer place and soothes our brain."[vii]

Dr. Susan Johnson

EFT guru

Often, when couples come for help on their relationship, and our client care manager, Melanie, asks them on the phone why they are coming, the response will be: they can't communicate. The couple wants to work on their communication.

It's funny to have couples ask for advice with "communication". Frequently, these are professionals that are highly capable and competent communicators in their role of physicians, lawyers, executives, line foreman, human resource manager, or executive assistant. Bakers, mechanics, accountants—all have to communicate to help their job go smoothly.

Highly capable individuals with an incredible capacity to express themselves attend marital therapy asking for help in communication. And they are right—when they attempt to speak to their spouse, they get defensive and non-productive. They watch themselves be hostile and self-protective, instead of collaborative. Spouses snap at their partner in a manner they wouldn't dream of doing at work. When they try to explain themselves, their capacity to articulate disappears and they stumble over their words. They can't even think to come up with helpful responses and instead observe nasty barbs explode out of their mouths towards their spouse in ways that would embarrass them if friends or colleagues were there to witness it.

There is an occasional couple that requires skill training to learn what it looks like to speak respectfully, how to inquire further about another person's opinion, and how to navigate a conflict. There are some that have never been around kind and gentle discussion that opens the door to productive dialogue. In those cases, skill building may be helpful.

However, what is much more often the case is that the connection between the couple is the issue. Once the connection is repaired, the communication ceases to become an issue. It's hard to communicate deeply and effectively with your spouse when you aren't sure your spouse has got your back.

***

I'm a science geek. I love to study things. To appreciate what works, and how it functions, and what we can learn from understanding our world better using scientific research.

We were created for relationships. We need relationships to survive. Relationships are as important to our health as oxygen, food, water and sunshine. Without relationships we suffer. In my 2018 Tedx talk, I said:

Julianne Holt-Lunstad's analysis of 148 studies found that people that have better social connections have a 50% reduced risk of early death. The risk of social isolation is comparable to smoking 15 cigarettes a day, and carries more risk than obesity or air pollution.

Strong bonds help cardiovascular health, strengthen immune response, keep brains sharp, and slows cellular aging.

Relationships are an integral part of mental health.

Robert Waldinger, the current head of Harvard Study of Adult Development, says that the clearest and most conclusive message that we get from this 80 year study is that: 'Good relationships keep us happier and healthier. Period.[viii]

Simply: **we require connection.**

***

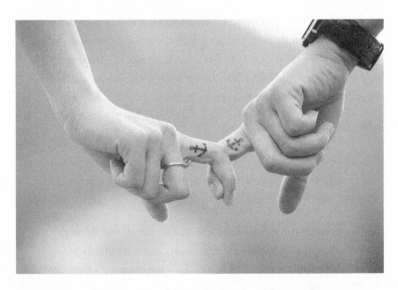

The anchors on those fingers? Yeah…being loved does that.

Feeling secure, knowing you belong—it anchors a person. And when an individual is securely anchored, it creates a sense of balance. Rather like when I learned to play basketball: feet shoulder width apart, knees slightly bent, weight over both feet, arms held up in front. This was known as the triple threat position. This balanced and anchored position puts a person in an optimal stance to pass, shoot or dribble.

Being loved in a meaningful relationship does that in our lives. We are better able to tackle challenges, have difficult conversations, and move forward effectively.

Our brains do better, we function better, we can solve problems better, and we move through the world more productively when we have meaningful, life-giving relationships in our lives. There are many scientific results that demonstrate that to us objectively and clearly.

***

We know that couples do better when they are connected. We all do better when we have meaningful connections with family and a few significant friends. Scientifically has measured and shown our lives are enhanced when we have people in our corner that are <u>A.R.E.</u>:

Accessibility:

I can reach you. When I need you, I can find you. You are there for me. Physical and emotional availability. When I need help, or reassurance, or simply want contact, I can trust you that you are there.

Responsive:

I can rely on you to hear me and respond When I say something, you respond. You let me know I matter. Your voice, your body language, your timing tells me you hear me and I am important to you.

Engaged:

You connect with me—meaningfully. I can tell you're in the conversation; that the relationship is something you're working at. You decrease my isolation and increase connection.

This is one step beyond available and responsive. You may be around to see me upset about my day, but if you tell me I'm silly and overreacting, you aren't engaged with my distress, I will feel disconnected from you,[ix]

Being available, responsive and engaged changes how we respond to our world. Husbands and wives that A.R.E. there for each other is a combination that is incredible.

We become more resilient, tolerant, creative, relaxed, energized, confident and capable.

The question husbands and wives need to ask is not: "Can we communicate?" but rather, "Are we connected?" Connected people can use the communication ability they had early in the relationship, and still have with friends and colleagues.

A.R.E. you connected as a couple?

8 SNICKERS AND LOVE MAPS

Over three years have passed since Jim and I have been married. I thought I knew Jim well. I found out recently, I've still got a few things to learn.

Our son got married to his sweetheart on a Saturday in her hometown. We travelled to this quaint little village by plane and then by car. The wedding occurred on a warm, sunny day. and they professed their love in front of family and friends overlooking the lake, with mountains in the distance. It was exquisite. Jim gave a terrific speech at the wedding. Overall–an awesome day. On Sunday, we flew home.

While we were waiting for our connection home in Vancouver, Husband ducked into a store to buy chocolate for the flight. We love chocolate!

An hour into the flight, I asked Jim to pull out the chocolate. As he reached for his backpack, he said, "I picked up my favorite kind."

And that was when I realized:

I wasn't sure what his favorite kind of chocolate was.

See, he generally purchases Reese's peanut butter cups. Because he knows it's my favorite.

As he was unzipping his bag, I'm frantically scrolling through the Rolodex of my memory to discover if I could come up with his favorite. I wanted to know I knew what he would pull out of the bag before I looked at it.

I couldn't.

Then he pulled out a small bag of Snickers bites.

Those Snickers surprised me.

I didn't like that sense of not knowing him well enough to identify that.

***

John Gottman speaks of the value of love maps.[x] A love map is an understanding of your partner's internal world.

It's about basic things like favorite foods, fond childhood memories; what they like to watch on Netflix and what is the most frustrating part of their job.

But it's far more than that. It's about knowing your spouse's dreams, goals, values, fears, joys and fundamental understanding of life.

Having a love maps is understanding who your spouse is by knowing all sorts of details about them:

***

Love maps are an excellent tool to love your partner better.

When I know what my husband's:

- favorite chocolate bar is, I can get it when I want to give him a treat.
- hot buttons are, I can carefully avoid them when we are having a heated discussion–that way we can stay on the topic, and I won't unnecessarily upset him.
- values are, I recognize when it makes sense to buy something spur of the moment because we will both agree on it, and when I will hold off until we discuss it and make a joint decision because he might feel differently. Collaboration is always a good idea when you don't see eye to eye.
- response to fatigue after a long, hard day of work, I can understand how best to be compassionate towards him, when he needs it.
- reaction will be to bad news, I perceive how to best react to him and give support to him.

Having a love map of a partner with many explicit details means I am better able to love my partner. He is better able to trust me because I realize how to "be there" for him more reliably. I can build trust in the smallest of moments because I have paid attention, and that attention to his preferences and style allows me to let him know all of that matters.

I can let him experience that he matters.

We do better in close relationships when we aren't just generically respectful and kind. To know the other person with enough specificity, we can show our love by having them experience being known and cared for.

Love is in the details.

9 THE HIDDEN DANGERS OF OVERFUNCTIONING

I hurt my back months ago. The physiotherapist said I likely ruptured a disc in my lower back. The resulting injury has resulted in more pain in my leg than in my back. This sciatic pain has been high for several months.

I went to visit a physiotherapist, Mike, who is a professor at a university. I met him when I taught there, and I like how he practices. As a systems therapist, I value when people work to notice an issue and then work beyond fixing the problem. To track back to discover where the problem arose—and then how it was that issue came about. When I've taken my sons to be treated by him, he has effectively fixed back problems by addressing the ankle, or knee problems by focusing on issues in the trunk.

As Mike is assessing my back a few weeks ago, he does a simple test. He has me lie on my tummy and lift one leg at a time off the plinth a few inches from the hip. I can do it—on my left and my right leg. I mean, it's a lot of work on my left side, and not as comfortable, but I can do it.

And he says: "AHHHH!", like he just learned something super

important.

Follow me carefully here.

To have me understand the significance of his discovery, he has me set my hand on my gluteal muscles (affectionately called "gluts" by those in the biz—the big chunky muscles in the butt) and says: "Touch your right butt cheek when you lift your right leg up".

I placed my hand on my right butt cheek...and my right glut tightens to elevate my leg. Normal.

He says, "Now, touch your left butt cheek when you lift your left leg up."

My leg goes up...but my left gluts stay soft. They stay squishy. (Sorry...too much information from a therapist?) It was weird to detect the marked difference in the way the muscle groups were acting.

And he explains: "Two muscle groups—the hamstrings [the muscles in the back of your legs] and the gluteal muscles should be sharing together in the effort of extending your leg up. The system is wonky on your left side and your hamstrings are doing *all* the work. Your gluts aren't firing on your left side when you raise your leg"

***

Mike then goes on to tell me what marriage counseling had long ago deeply ingrained in me:

When one part underfunctions, the whole thing can still function *if another part over functions.*

He told me the implications of the pairing of an over functioning muscle group with an under functioning muscle group for my body.

Mike didn't actually need to tell me.

I could have given him the lecture.

Because I've seen marriages die with this pattern never being addressed.

When one part underfunctions and then another part over functions to compensate, it pulls the relationship out of alignment. And being out of alignment creates all sorts of related issues.

It works...but *at a price*. Pain. Decreased strength. Fatigue.

***

My recent back injury taught me about the pain and discomfort when one set of muscles under function and another collection of muscles compensate to overfunction.

Underfunctioners often don't recognize that they are underfunctioning. They aren't awake in their life. They don't understand others are looking after the practical and emotional demands in the world around them. They may also not realize the long-term cost of allowing a partner in life/work/friendship to do most/all the effort. Underfunctioning is a relationship killer.

But—drum roll please: Overfunctioning is also a relationship killer.

***

The majority of us grow up believing that being kind is a good thing.

And it is.

But kindness that robs others of their ability to fulfill their roles in the world that is *not kind*.

That's *enablement*.

***

Overfunctioning is treating someone as if they can't do it for themselves.

It's saying, "I don't trust you to fold your laundry, so I'll do it".

Overfunctioning is disrespectful.

It's saying, "I can't see your abilities or trust them. Move over and I'll do it."

Overfunctioning is dismissive.

It's saying, "I don't believe you are capable of paying for this yourself, so, of course I'll buy it for you," or "I will agree with you that you don't need to participate. I won't make us both uncomfortable by insisting you to show up in our lives. The kids and I can live our lives without you."

In essence, "You're not that important or competent…I can do without you."

Overfunctioning is dis-empowering.

It's taking away that feeling from someone. You know, that feeling—that rush that happens when you work hard and git'er done. That spirit of doing your job right. That sense of, "I don't feel like it, but I'll have that significant but awkward conversation with our teenager, because I can contribute". That notion of, "It was hard. Really hard. And I got it done!" Gosh that feeling is good. That "I can put my head down on my pillow peacefully tonight for a job well done today" feeling. That, "Whew, that was brave and hard and scary, but I DID IT!!" feeling.

Overfunctioners rob underfunctioners.

They teach their loved ones—the underfunctioners, that they are incapable, not-good-enough, and simply not competent.

Oh, overfunctioners don't express these ideas in words, at all. They don't even think it in their heads. Matter of fact, most overfunctioners will be horrified to learn this. They may not recognize it. They work to be benevolent.

But trust me, overfunctioners will read this. The whole thing. It's in their nature.

They can't help it!

***

A friend of mine, a lovely woman, came by her overfunctioning honestly.

I love her.

It was a natural result from her survival strategies, which were actually adaptive for her in her life. She was a perfectionist. Her overfunctioning/perfectionistic strategies were the way to survive in a home that had an alcoholic parent. It created a modicum of organization in a world that she found chaotic and unpredictable.

So, now as an adult, she did all the laundry folding while he watched the game. He didn't mind being able to focus on the television. She loved that all the corners were lined up on the towels. She fed the dog, because then she knew Trixie wasn't being overfed. She bought the groceries, and put them away in exacting order, and cleaned the bathroom, just so. Everything—all the rest of the house, just perfect. I could go on. If she did it, she was confident it was done right. She liked the sense of doing it herself so she could ensure it all met her standards.

And then, over the years, she became a ball of resentment because she was exhausted—and her husband was still watching the game.

He was happy—until he saw that she wasn't happy. He was a great guy, really. Just blithely clueless until the moment she announced, "Enough".

He agreed to go to therapy.

When they showed up for counseling, she learned over time to turn to her husband during the course of the week, and in a very deliberate (and humorous, really) manner, to turn directly to face him, and would say: "I AM DROPPING THE BALL!" With her hands, she would mimic the action of dropping the ball.

That was the hint he needed to "pick up the ball" and look around. Fold the laundry. Make supper. Clean up the kitchen.

He actually needed some coaching to wake up and notice, at first. She rather trained the *looking around* right out of him.

This wasn't just about getting him to do more chores. Nope, by that time, chores were the least of their worries.

See, the problems were far beyond basic tasks like emptying the dishwasher. She was overfunctioning *in every area* of their relationship.

She was ensuring that their world worked in just about every respect. She knew what his favorite restaurants were and made reservations at those places, including she spent less so he could spend more, she placated him in arguments, and generally invested more in their lives than he was.

And that wasn't healthy for anybody.

As they continued therapy, and she functioned less, he could pick up some slack.

This whole process wasn't without its challenges—scary, anxious moments.

She wondered what would happen if she chose to go out and leave him to make dinner for the children.

The therapist suggested he would make a meal. Like a capable adult.

Or he wouldn't.

He needed to understand what happened when he didn't make dinner. It would be uncomfortable for him and this would likely irk her. A normal response to someone goofing up. And they would deal with it.

Natural outcomes.

He needed to be trusted to function. He wasn't incapable.

He needed:

- to be given permission to fail,
- an opportunity to figure out what needed to get done
- to do it his way, and
- the space to actively participate in the relationship.

***

Picture this: 2 people standing in a canoe.

Tippy image, isn't it?

Both need to be attuned to the actions of others to keep the canoe balanced. If one leans out one direction, even a little, the other needs to lean the other way to keep it stabilized.

If one leans out a lot, the other leans out a lot the other way...and the canoe stays stable.

The canoe won't tip if the two are leaning way out in different directions, as long as they balance each other out.

The canoe is stable. It's not tipping. And the two in the canoe stay dry—they aren't in the water.

But they sure ain't comfortable.

And it probably isn't sustainable.

And ultimately, the canoe is at greater risk of capsizing. It's exhausting to ensure the boat doesn't tip by leaning so far out to match the other.

It's. Just. Plain. Hard.

The underfunctioning/overfunctioning dynamic is a partnership just like that.

We can over function with children, with co-workers and friends—and husbands.

Overfunctioners work super hard. They do so much generally with the best intentions—consciously. They do what they do at personal cost to benefit the greater good.

The advantages to overfunctioning aren't conscious.

Overfunctioners also receive advantages from their behavior that are beyond their conscious awareness.

Overfunctioners get to:

- feel like a hero...like they are rescuing folks who need them desperately. If they keep someone in their lives at less than full capacity, they get feel good about themselves. Who doesn't love to be a rescuer?

- control their world. How many of us haven't done all the labor of the group project at school because then we were confident we would get the A?

Overfunctioning:

- is the ultimate in quality control.
- provides an effective strategy to reduce or even avoid conflict. If you do everything, there's no need to argue about it, with anybody.
- is a safe way to *keep peace*. No challenging required.
- ensures you are needed. If you train people to require you, then they can't leave you. It might even make it hard for them to be mad at you. Being needed means you are pseudo-secure in the relationship

As much as overfunctioners resent the role and complain about it...they can refuse to give it up.

Equalizing the relationship requires brave conversations and courageous self-awareness. It means holding space for uncertainty and discomfort.

Choosing to leave old painful but familiar ruts leaves room for establishing new ways of being together.

10 THE HIDDEN COST OF UNDERFUNCTIONING

It stands to reason that with every overfunctioner, there is an underfunctioner.

As I mentioned in the last chapter, Mike, my physiotherapist, found that one set of muscles was not firing as he was working on my back. He wanted to work with me to solve the dysfunctional muscle pattern of one muscle group doing the work of two muscle groups while the second one took a holiday.

My body was out of alignment. It was making my back pain worse. There were many related issues.

The **over/underfunctioning works**...but at a *huge price*. Pain. Decreased strength. Fatigue.

***

The solution, as Mike told me, was profound:

The strategy to fix the underfunctioning/overfunctioning dysfunction is **to get the under functioning muscles to start firing.**

So, Mike taught me to work to first deliberately tighten my left butt cheek and then lift my left leg. I had to reteach the muscles that weren't working how to get involved again.

The way to fixing this was to remind those underfunctioning muscles to do their share, with awareness and repetition and practice and strengthening.

It was weird.

I had to "find" the muscle and figure out what signals to send to it to get it to contract.

Not that those muscles didn't want to work—it was more like they had forgotten how.

It wasn't easy at first.

But even after two sets of 10 in the office on that visit, those gluts were already starting to begin to do what they were supposed to do.

I do this exercise every evening now before I go to bed. My left gluts still only work about 80-90% of what the right side can do.

But this, combined with the other exercises Mike has given me meant marked improvement. In the past week, I have slept through the night without pain medication for the first time in months.

Fixing this under/overfunctioning pattern in my gluts and hamstrings has literally changed my daily life.

***

Underfunctioners rarely realize that they are underfunctioning— they just aren't awake in their life. They don't realize others are looking after the practical and emotional demands in the world around them. They may also not realize the long-term cost of allowing a partner in life/work/friendship to do most/all the work.

They may not understand how their underfunctioning is a relationship killer.

***

Underfunctioner—take note:

You've likely never heard of underfunctioning. You likely wouldn't trouble yourself to look it up.

Chances are you are reading this because your spouse says it's super important for you to read.

If so, consider it a gift?

It might seem easier to let your spouse regularly do the cleanup. It might be a convenient excuse to say you suck at folding laundry. You might beg off grocery shopping or driving the kids because you're tired and you've worked hard.

And underfunctioning isn't just about chores, ok? It's also easier and less vulnerable to not start hard conversations or invest in sharing your heart. You might just choose to not start a conversation—turning the television on is easier. You may not get around to check in on her, not find out what is or isn't working for her. There are many ways you may not be holding up your end of the relationship.

There are some significant short-term perks to being an underfunctioner.

And your spouse may well pick up the slack, even with an attempt to be understanding.

It might help to know overfunctioners are willing to over function quite a long time...because:

- it's easier to do it than explain and invite you to take part. It's an uncomfortable conversation to tell someone they aren't stepping up
- they come from a world where one parent overfunctioned while the other underfunctioned and it's all they know
- they have explained and cajoled and argued and you have blown them off...and they have given up on you

However, marriages where one spouse is consistently underfunctioning while the other one overfunctions are at serious risk. This dynamic creates an atmosphere of resentment and distance. This pattern sets the tone where disengagement is very possible.

The sad thing with the dynamic of an overfunctioning/underfunctioning marriage is that it limps along, with everything getting done and everything mostly looking ok— until one day, the overfunctioner can't do it anymore.

The marriage has been silently eroding for ages and can seem to collapse overnight.

Marriages function best when the two work together to find a rhythm that works for both partners—when they work in tandem.

Underfunctioner, if your significant other has troubled you to read this chapter, would you be willing to recognize yourself in it? Would you be willing to acknowledge that your partner is struggling under the weight of overfunctioning now?

You as an underfunctioner could pay the ultimate price of losing someone you really care about—if not in body, then in spirit. Being able to watch the game while she runs around getting things done might seem like a good deal. Ultimately, however, you **both** will pay the price.

If your significant other has had you read this chapter, would you be willing to begin an uncomfortable-but-ultimately-beneficial discussion of curiosity? Could you ask lots of questions and reserve your reactions, just to really hear the experience of the overfunctioner in your life?

Would you be willing to notice that you are at serious risk of losing the most important relationship in your life? Because you benignly choose to omit seeing how much harder your spouse works at your relationship than you, your spouse is building resentment in a dangerous way? Would you be willing to explore this?

This isn't just about housework--making supper, laundry, emptying the dishwasher (though it is that too).

This is about:

- Engaging with the kids,
- Starting conversations with your wife about what she is interested in
- Helping with homework
- Pulling out the calendar and being the one to insert the kid's schedules on it
- About raising the conversation of your unresolved last argument to actually pursue its end
- Taking initiative to write the birthday card to your mother this year (and buying it ahead of time!)
- Arranging the Friday night date this time
- Saying, "I love you" first, not just, "I love you too" in response
- Being the one to plan a special glass of something at the end of the day

When the underfunctioner, as hard as it can be to get more involved, finds a way to engage, it releases the overfunctioner. (Sometimes you may even need to gently kick the overfunctioner in the butt, as in, "Stop doing all the work and then resenting me for it. I want to share in the work of our lives. Trust me enough to not do it all yourself").

It frees everyone to a marriage that has a good chance of working well.

11 EMOTIONAL LABOR

My husband, Jim, spent a week in Texas in the fall working with a team to rebuild a house destroyed in a hurricane. He has a seasonal business, and that frees him up for stuff like this. I was happy to have him go use his skills to help others.

I was solo parenting our youngest high school aged son during his absence. At one point, this son asked me to text his coach to ask about an upcoming practice.

I realized I couldn't text the coach because I didn't have the coach's contact information.

Jim does all the thinking, planning, marking on the calendar, negotiating car pool for this son's sports activities. I help with driving, I love to watch him play, I'll register him for a program, but I'm not the *point person* for his sports. I help out in ways Jim asks me to help.

When we got married, and were figuring out who would do what, we decided that he would be the coordinator of this boy's activities. Jim had been doing it before our marriage, and we felt it made sense for him to continue.

While my husband gone, I had to figure a few things out that aren't normally my department.

Later in the same week, when a friend dropped by, she handed me a fistful of mail from our mailbox. I usually come in the back door, and so rarely check or bring in the mail. Once again: Jim's department. I hadn't even realized that the mail wasn't coming in the house because it's not on my radar.

My husband does it.

All the time.

When Jim came home from his week of building, I had a whole new appreciation for all the little things he does. I realized that I rarely look after making sure we have milk in the fridge. Husband looks after the noticing, and then one of us buys it when he says it's time.

I had to make coffee each morning—Jim does that, too.

While Jim was with the team in Texas, they had no television and so they spent the evenings playing games and visiting. Husband noticed the richness and has suggested this week to turn off the television and talk. The quality of our relationship is on his radar.

Isn't that beautiful?

There are dozens of little ways that Jim helps our house hum along. I'm so grateful that Jim shares the *emotional labor* of our home.

***

Emotional labor is a term few are familiar with. Yet, by now, I suspect you have one of two reactions:

1. I know exactly what you mean, and all of that is exhausting and challenging. It takes up a lot of mental space but I do it so

automatically that sometimes I forget that I'm doing it. And then, I catch myself sometimes and think: "No wonder I'm so frazzled and overwhelmed".

2.   Oh, that stuff. Yeah, it's not something that's on my radar. It's really not such a big deal is it? I mean, how hard could it be?

Jim was a single dad when I met him. He learned, and he will tell you it was often the hard way, all the things that his late wife, Car, looked after. There was the time, in the months after he was widowed, when he went to pick up his youngest from school and he couldn't find him anywhere. There was a tense 90 minutes while he phoned every place he could think of to find this boy. Turns out another mom took him along with her boy to the birthday party of a good friend from school. Jim hadn't taken notice of the invitation, the date, the transportation, or the gift to give the birthday child. This wasn't anything he had every done before, while his wife was alive.

He had no choice but to figure out emotional labor on his own—and then do it.

While Jim was in Texas, I had the wonderful realization, in a felt sense, of what I had always intuitively known:

Jim shares the emotional labor of our household.

I am grateful.

***

Emotional labor has traditionally fallen to women. Historically, it wasn't just looking after the family calendar, and making sure everybody had what they needed to have, knew where to go and how to get there, and kept the whole house running smoothly, and coordinating with the community center, the school, the church/mosque/synagogue, etc.

Emotional labor also included being responsible for the husband's mental health and self-esteem by tasks such as not pursuing a meaningful career, ensuring that she appeared less intelligent than her husband, being helpless at the appropriate moments to ensure he could play the hero.

We would all like to think this part of emotional labor is only historical, but the vestiges remain and are noticed if you ask yourself some questions and then dig deep for answers.

When I speak with women, I still hear bits and pieces of, "Wives make the lives of their husbands work well," in a way that men, while still wanting to be kind to their wives, do not expect of themselves. For example, when I ask a woman why she doesn't tell her husband she is enraged by all the ways she feels taken for granted, she will simply say, "I don't want to hurt his feelings".

Do men say this as well? Absolutely. But, to be honest, there is a hesitancy by women I don't as often see in men to bring up topics that will likely upset their mates.

Historically, women are the ones that are to make the marriage, family, and household work--and, also, do it so that no one even notices all the things.

***

Emotional Labor includes:

- being the thoughtful one that looks after the other's wellbeing at the expense of oneself
- sensing what the one's spouse needs and wants and doing what it takes to bring the other satisfaction and psychological safety
- monitoring external relationships with family and friends, ensuring that others feel connected to you

and your family through visits, cards, family
gatherings, birthday parties, phone calls, and texts
- monitoring and maintaining the family calendar by
  scheduling the family activities by registering for
  programs; communicating with coaches, car pools
  and babysitters;
- naming family and marital challenges; doing research
  on these challenges online, with professionals,
  talking to friends; and gathering resources and
  possible strategies; and figuring out action plans
  for these challenges. This can range from figuring
  how how to transition an infant to solid foods,
  worrying about a child's rash, noticing distance in
  the marriage, figuring out why an adolescent is
  sullen and quiet and a thousand more.
- keeping tabs on the house, such as:
    o where the laundry is at—what loads
      require washing, drying, and folding,
    o determine needed groceries,
    o when the toilet and the rest of the
      bathroom has last been cleaned,
    o if the dishwasher needs emptying
    o and so on and so on and so on

Emotional labor is being the **quarter back** of the household. It is
knowing what is going on in every area of every person and every
part of the house and making sure it all gets looked after.

To be sure, the quarterback needs a team to give him time to
prepare the play, to pass off to, to catch the ball. The quarterback
plays because he loves the game, and he plays the game with his
team.

But being the quarterback of the household is exhausting. It's not
just implementing what needs doing, it is scanning the
environment: the children and the household and the calendar and

the fridge and the dishwasher and the washing machine and the carpool and the email and the marriage and the stress level and the season and the upcoming stuff and so on and so on—all the time.

***

Being the quarterback of the team is a lot of work.

Marriage in the twenty-first century with busy lives isn't meant to be a football game.

With busy lives, dual-career families, car-pooling, and the way we arrange playdates for our children these days, marriage is best seen as a soccer game. Where the ball gets passed back and forth, seamlessly. In soccer there are positions of defender and half-back and forward. Players have different roles and tasks, but they all take part fluidly, each taking the lead at different times.

Marriage, is best collaborative, sharing the role of where the ball goes. People having various areas of specialty where they excel and are comfortable, but the relationships is reciprocal and collaborative. The ball of emotional labor gets passed back and forth.

***

In many relationships, the female in the relationship does the majority of the emotional labor. Historically, perhaps there was logic to it. Now...not so much.

The important and not-so-obvious thing about emotional labor is this: *Emotional labor is almost entirely invisible.*

I wasn't fully aware of all the things Jim does to make our lives work until he went out of town. (And I suspect, he picks up on all the things I get done when I am out of town and not available to do them.)

Most of us don't know—in fact, we can't know, all the emotional labor our spouse does unless we talk about it.

Sometimes, it's even hard to talk about it. So... I made it a little easier. I created an informal, fun quiz intended as a starting point for a discussion on emotional labor.

***

Emotional Labor Quiz

Give one point in the appropriate column:

(Suggestion: Copy this and ask your spouse to complete it and compare answers. It would be a great discussion!)

You	Your partner	
		The one is more likely to know how much milk is in your fridge
		The one who knows when it is time to invite your parents/aunt and uncle/elderly friend over
		Which one of you most recently looked at the other to ask: "how are we really doing as a couple?"
		The one who knows the most urgent "fix it" tasks in the household and holds those tasks on a list on their head

		When going out for dinner, the one who is more likely to say, "Let's go where you want to go!" or "You pick!"
		After your last disagreement as a couple, the person who first approached the other to gently reconnect
		The one who puts most events on the family calendar
		If you both have an important function on Friday night you need to attend together, the one is more likely to acquiesce, saying: "We'll do your thing."
		The one whose job it is to ensure the laundry is caught up and done (note: this differs from the one actually doing it)
		The one who is the Christmas shopping coordinator: getting Christmas lists, organizing the shopping, knows which boxes on the list are not yet checked, and most feels the pressure to ensure all that all shopping gets completed
		The one to arrange and/or cancel the babysitter/housekeeper/dog walker
		The one to notice that it is time for a "date night" out as a couple
		The one who sends the condolence cards and/or flowers when a person close to the family is grieving a death

		The one who is more likely to say to the other: "You've got a busy day tomorrow. You go to bed and I'll take care of what's left to do."
		The one who will know where that cord is for the rarely-used device that needs charging
		For parents of children under 18:
		The one to notice that your child is struggling and could use a little extra tender loving care
		If a note needs writing for school, or a permission slip needs signing, the one is likely to take care of it
		The one who is more likely to research issues your child is facing to develop strategies to address the problem
		The person who planned the date and the invitations for your child's birthday party
		The one who figures out which clothes are needed as the child grow, which still fit from last summer, when the child needs new shoes etc.
		The person who bought the birthday gift for the last birthday party your child attended (with or without your child along)
		The last person to have talked to your child's coach/piano teacher, etc.

		The one who knows where to locate your child's immunization records
		The one most likely to get up when your child has a nightmare and is frightened.
		The person who is more likely to do the juggling of schedules to stay home when your child is ill and stays home from school/daycare.
Total:	Total:	The greater the disparity between the total of your two scores, the greater the load of emotional labor falls to one spouse

Subtract 3 points from your score if, when your spouse expresses frustration, your answer often involves something like: "Give me a list, and I'm happy to help."

Subtract 3 more points from your score if, in the last two weeks, you have done something and then deliberately pointed it out to your spouse to *show off* the fruits of your labor. (e.g. "I cleaned the kitchen for you, did you notice? Doesn't it look great?")

***

To simply blame the person who does little emotional labor in a couple isn't fair. Pointing a finger at one person doesn't recognize the complexity of the situation: the culture we live in, the development of patterns over time, and the mechanisms in place that perpetuate the continuation of the cycle.

The ironic part of carrying the majority of the emotional labor is that: The unwritten job description of the role of the person who carries the burden of emotional labor also includes a mandate to not complain about it, or notice it, or mention it—ever. Included in the unstated code of emotional laborer is to do it quietly.

The only time the burden of emotional labor comes out is during an argument.

This is when the Person Bearing the Emotional Labor (PBEL) has the: Dreaded Meltdown (DM). The DM comes out as a litany of complaints that seem petty and banal, quite out of proportion to whatever is happening at the moment. The DM comes out loud and long. It feels like an undeserved barrage of negativity. Frequently, though not always, there will be tears.

Almost inevitably, the Person who Does Not Bear the Emotional Labor (PDNBEL) gets defensive. Because the over-reaction to the single laundry basket in the hallway, or the lack of whole milk in the fridge, or that the sympathy card left on the hallway table is left unsigned and mailed seems "bat-sh*t crazy".

I hack into people's lives for a living. I know how this goes. When the PBEL unloads a torrent of seemingly petty concerns after they leave a sock on the floor or something that seems equally trivial, the PDNBEL, says exasperatedly (or even kindly): "Give me a list and I'll help you."

Usually, the PDNBEL is actually kind and caring, maybe confused—and genuinely wants the ugliness to end. To bring sanity to the situation, and in an effort to be kind and sympathetic and make it all better even though it seems completely unnecessary, because the PBEL seems utterly ridiculous, the PDNBEL offers the most obvious, very kind and very noble gesture. Assistance by asking for a list seems like a good thing.

While a spouse (statistically, a husband) intends this to be well meaning, it exactly illustrates and compounds the problem.

On some occasions, the PBEL will describe items for a list with some relief, desperate to have things off that mental "to-do" list.

However, most often, to the sheer confusion of the PDNBEL, when they offer to work on things on a list they request...it does not go well. At all.

Often, though, that line meets with complete exasperation.

The line, "Give me a list and I'll help you," though said with genuine care, perpetuates the problem. The PBEL still manages the list, still carries responsible for the carrying out of the list, and now will only get assistance with all that they are feeling responsible for. The PBEL still carries the burden.

Sharing emotional labor means saying: "I will take on some of this load as mine. It's not your responsibility to carry it all."

This is important: We've learned that a husband doesn't babysit his children. Mostly, this way of thinking has disappeared in the last quarter century or so. We know that a father looks after his children, parents his children, or spends the evening with his children—but doesn't "babysit" his children.

Similarly, a partner doesn't help empty the dishwasher or help out by buying the sympathy card. A partner simply shares in the duties and tasks of the household.

***

Jim will tell you, if you visit with him, of the time he stepped around the laundry basket of clean laundry that his late wife, Car, put on the stairs early in their marriage.

Car wanted to see how long it would take Jim to notice it and do something about the clean laundry. She had washed, dried and folded it. Would he automatically take part in the last step of the laundry by putting it away?

He walked up and down those stairs for days, moving to the side to avoid the basket. Completely unawares he was doing so.

After about 5 days, she gave up and had a conversation with him about it. She addressed it head on. Car decided not to be silently resentful and quietly overburdened. I don't know if there was a Dreaded Meltdown involved or not.

She invited Husband to become informed about what he hadn't noticed.

Husband has never forgotten this.

He tells the story with a chuckle, but make no mistake. He has remembered the lesson and lives a different life because of it.

Because, here's the thing: A person doesn't know what they don't know. A person can't know what they don't know.

Notice how "Will you work with me on this?" differs from, "Will you help me with this?" It's a move from being in charge to being a collaborator.

***

Emotional labor is the intangible effort that goes into keeping life afloat.

It isn't just knowing that your kid is struggling in math. It's:

- understanding why there is a struggle.
- talking to others and looking online for several strategies to address it
- problem solving how to afford the strategy that makes sense
- bringing it up with your spouse in a way to get the spouse onboard

- figuring out how to talk to your child about the struggle in a way that reduces anxiety and increases self confidence, and only then,
- having the conversation with the child

So many chunks of emotional labor have multiple pieces to each of them.

There is so much of emotional labor that can go unnoticed that even the one doing it may not realize.

***

Imagine how much stronger marriages would be if PBEL wasn't overwhelmed and frustrated. Imagine how much richer the marriage would be if the PDNBEL invested in the hidden layers of effort required to keep the household alive?

Imagine the intimacy gained by having the awkward but courageous conversations to find out all the ways your partner invests in which you would have no awareness?

Henry Ford said, "Coming together is a beginning, staying together is progress, and working together is a success."

This working together isn't easy, but it is worth it.

12 10 RULES OF EMOTIONAL ENGAGEMENT

Jim and I love each other, but we don't always see eye to eye. We have to sort out disagreement and differences of opinion and perceived and actual slights just like anybody else. I don't like it when Husband and I are at odds with each other.

My world isn't entirely right when Jim and I aren't right.

And when he and I are solid, I move along in my day in a more solid way. I value when I know he and I are on the same page; when I know he's got my back and we're good.

But—here's the thing: I believe in hashing it out. I don't like ignoring the underlying tension hoping the trouble will disappear on its own.

I don't feel comfortable with a fragile ceasefire existence where we are ignoring an issue to appear that we're OK. I've worked with enough couples to know pretending something isn't there, doesn't make it not there.

The instability and uncertainty of ignored stuff will show up sinisterly in different ways in our relationship as we go about our lives. I don't feel comfortable living with the subtle effects of untended bits of relationship debris.

I want a relationship where we're actually good with each other, which means taking care of the crap as it comes up, to make us stronger. It means welcoming the tension of a conflict as a deliberate lifestyle.

I don't love conflict with Jim, but I do find it *less worse* than not dealing with the conflict.

***

Jim and I, formally and informally, have developed guidelines around our conflict. We've worked at this, explicitly and implicitly over time to develop a style of conflict that is authentic about the tension and the upset. However, we have worked towards working through that conflict in a style that doesn't create all sorts of damage that needs healing later.

One of the big dangers of working out a conflict is to incur further damage during the conflict itself.

Just as a bell can't be unrung, nasty words uttered in the intensity of the moment can't be unsaid, and can't be unheard.

I frequently work with couples who come in not only process a major marital issue, but the added fallout of the fights that have arisen during the processing of the issue.

***

Collateral damage of unacceptable behaviour during an argument stings. Even when everyone calms down, and there is huge regret for the actions it still hurts. Threatening divorce or calling a partner names is something people often regret later. (If they can even remember that they did it while they were all fired up!) However, it sticks in a partner's head and creates distance. That distance shows up on the couch when you're watching TV later. It is then that small irritations that wouldn't usually matter start to matter.

***

I hate messing up when I'm dysregulated and upset. I know that when I'm mad at Jim, and/or when I'm feeling like he's mad at me, I am not nearly at my best. I dislike knowing I've acted outside of my values in the heat of the moment. Because of that, we have ground rules that minimize the damage that occurs during the argument.

There are things we don't say, lines we have decided ahead of time we don't go past:

Lines. We. Will. Not. Cross.

We **all** have lines we don't cross in arguments. Some folks say, "I'm not in control of what happens when I'm upset, so don't hold it against me." Think about how often you have pulled a knife on your spouse, slugged your partner, or not done any number of outrageous and illegal things. See? *Of course* you don't cross some lines. Of course you have some ground rules you don't break.

I think the challenge is for us to be deliberate and conscious about the lines we do not cross. While calling your partner a "#*&%@^" may not be illegal, it can be almost impossible to come back from the heart wounding that is created by name calling.

The *lines that will not be crossed* are best clearly established at a time of calm; when you are fully connected to your best self and are clear on your values.

And it's not enough to decide not to cross them. Unless there are healthy alternatives in place that are known and understood, it's not realistic to expect those decisions will actually be honored in the heat of the moment.

***

I asked Jim what he thought our rules of engagement are, to see if our understandings matched.

This was our list of rules of engagement:

1. Comment about behaviors, not character. That means no calling names, which is labelling a person.
2. We work to own our feelings and our concerns with "I" language. Blaming with "you" language is not considered helpful. E.g. "I felt embarrassed when..." rather than, "You embarrassed me when..."
3. Words like "never" and "always" are inflammatory...we try not to use superlatives that are extreme. This, by extension, means not using the ultimate superlative. We will never threaten the end of our marriage. That's just *mean*—a hollow threat that would do untold damage. If it ever would be uttered, there would have to be very serious grounds that made it possible or even probable.
4. Thinking is actually brilliant, and we have to allow space for thinking. In other words, silence can be a productive part of arguments. This one is important for me to remember because Husband is thoughtful and words come slower for him than me. If I'm not deliberate, I'll fill the spaces with my words in ways that aren't helpful. (Sometimes I will say with a wink, "If this is a dialogue, then it's your turn. I'm not sure what you're thinking.") I have to remember to not do all the talking, with filling up the empty spaces.
5. When we start going in circles, or one of us becomes too upset, either of us has permission to take a break. One lets the other know it isn't working, and we say

something like, "We matter too much for me to keep going and say something I will regret later. I need space." It helps when the one left behind knows that the one taking a break is not rejecting or abandoning...just protecting the relationship.

6. When one of us takes a break, we resume after a break and finish talking it through--an hour later, or after the kids go to bed, or the next day. That sometimes means falling asleep with things left unsettled if one or both of us is too tired to be productive in the conversation. In that case, it means remembering we are OK even when we are not OK. Sort of like remembering in the middle of a flu that even though it feels like you're gonna die, you will get better. It's important to hold on to the deeper truth, and not get carried away by the moment's feeling.

7. We allow ourselves the ability to say, "I'm too tired to give this conversation justice." We need to do it another time. We will often check in, "There's something I want to run by you. Is now a good time?" Just because I'm not up for hearing him in the moment, does not mean I don't care. I'm glad he can hold that.

8. We give each other and ourselves room to be stupid and to own it. Even in the intensity of our anger, we try to not take ourselves too seriously. It's not uncommon for one of us, in the middle of an argument to say something like: "I get I'm being unreasonable and not fair but...". Or, "I will have a clearer grasp on this tomorrow, but right now I'm very upset that...". Or, "I know you probably didn't mean it this way, but the story I'm telling myself is that you...". Or, "What I just said wasn't kind, and I'm trying hard to be sorry, but I don't know how else to say it". It's brutally kind honesty at a deep level even when we're upset.

9. *This is not our first rodeo.* We know the other's hot buttons. We know where each other is most vulnerable, and where the most tender spots are—and are careful to not only *not exploit* them, but take extra care. For example, Jim knows that trust is legitimately fragile for me because of a previous relationship. He doesn't overreact when I'm upset around a trust issue, and he's careful to reassure me. Similarly, I know that if I mention certain things to him in an argument, it's nothing but a low blow. He will never deserve that.

10. We argue knowing that we got into this marriage because we truly care for and love each other. Hold on to that truth, however hard, throughout the discussion. Act out of this profound and real truth, even if you feel differently in the moment. Sometimes, holding onto this big picture isn't easy—but it's always worth it.

***

Underneath it all, simply is this: **I trust that my husband is for my good, not my harm.** When he says or does something that feels hurtful, I work to remember the big picture. And he words to trust that I ultimately have his back, and I am for his good.

The big picture is this:

We love each other.

We will have our moments of selfishness, self-preservation, and downright goofs. But the fundamental core is: *we are a team.* We picked this relationship and are invested in making it work. The small acts of caring, consideration and love throughout the week reinforce this. We work, imperfectly to be sure, to have love permanence. I want to remember that even when I'm furious with Husband (and I have been!), ultimately he loves me.

I work hard to remember that he doesn't have it as a core goal to be a jerk to me. On occasion, that becomes a mantra in my head: *"Jim is fundamentally not a jerk."* Over and over, to temper my reaction. That sounds perfectly obvious now to me as I write this. However, there are moments of anger where it needs to be a deliberate choice to repeat and believe this line. My mind, when I'm threatened, can become almost convinced that he is deliberately being a jerk to me. My brain plays tricks on me when I'm mad. Yours, too, right?

Often, figuring out how to help a couple hold on to the thought that, "We are ultimately for each other's good, not harm," is the key to successful therapy with that couple.

***

There is one more fundamental agreement we've made in our relationship:

If either one of us says we need to go see a marriage therapist, the other one must cooperate with the process.

No exceptions.

Statistically, it is more likely that Jim will pull the trigger on seeing a therapist.

Here's the deal: I work with words and conversations and relationship dynamics for a living. I know my way around a marital conflict like nobody's business. It's my job. We have discussed the possibility that without my realizing it, I could talk him out of his feelings or work my way out of a situation in a way that is not cool. This disadvantage he has because I am a professional relationship expert means that our relationship could become unfair for him and I might not even be aware. He might not even really understand what is happening—he'd just know it wasn't good. I so wouldn't want that.

I want Jim to love our relationship. I hope that if I am doing something destructive without being aware of it, that he will call me on it, on his own, or with the help of a therapist.

If either one of us feel:

- in over our head,
- that we repeatedly aren't heard,
- that something critical in our relationship is missing and our efforts to figure it out are unsuccessful,
- that something isn't working, and none of our efforts are effective to get it working again,

then we will both go to a therapist together.

Even if we:

- don't want to go
- are embarrassed
- think it's silly

We will go because our relationship will be more important than our desire to not go to a therapist.

***

I watch my kids play volleyball, basketball, soccer, baseball, badminton and any other number of sports. What makes these games not only fun to play, but also safe are the rules of the game, and the boundaries of the court. People know what they can do to play competitively, and what is illegal and qualifies for a foul or a penalty. The rules are necessary to ensure that there are less injuries, less disagreements, and more opportunity to simply enjoy the game.

Why don't you and your spouse write down your rules for disagreements? Figure them out. It might be an interesting conversation! Write them down and check them from time to time to see if they still fit for you, or if one needs to be changed or added. Find ways of making disagreements safer to discuss. Create ways to create engagement that seems messy at times, but doesn't become completely chaotic. Develop a structure that will free you both up to better be able to discuss topics that would otherwise be avoided.

13 THE IMPERCEPTIBLE, AMOST IRRESISTABLE SLIDE INTO INFIDELITY

I've worked extensively with couples in the immediate, devastating, agonizing aftermath of the discovery of an affair.

It's hard to watch the couple come in. One spouse, whose world has been rocked at its very foundations has puffy eyes, a huge lostness, feeling their life is suddenly very different. There's generally a wildness about their eyes, with a frantic wondering: "What else don't I know?".

The other partner, the unfaithful, is often contrite, with poor eye contact. Their shoes receive a lot of careful examination. It does something to a person to violate their own moral code in a manner in which they have limited understanding.

One of the especially hard parts for the cheating partner is to observe the agony of their partner. It is its own special little hell to witness the one you have committed your life to loving be in complete devastation as the result of your choices. It's excruciating to watch someone you love be in such pain knowing you caused it.

For many couples, we take a two pronged approach when they come in to work through infidelity:

1. The *infidelity is a problem* of betrayal that requires healing work
2. The *infidelity is a symptom* of a problem. It exposes a susceptibility between the couple or within one of the partners that created circumstances ripe for an affair to develop. This requires relationship repair work. Cheating is hard on a marriage, and it's tough coming back from its discovery—but it's possible to develop a marriage that is stronger and more vibrant than before the affair. The affair can be a cue that either or both of you has work to do in area of the exposed vulnerability.

There is a style of affair that is difficult for couples to wrap their head around. The one that develops organically, so imperceptibly that it seems impossible to recognize when it started. And then seems inconceivable to stop once it has begun.

***

Ever heard of the frog in the kettle? It's an apt picture…

If you plop a frog in a pot of piping hot water—it immediately recognizes the discomfort and danger and promptly hops out.

If you put a frog in a saucepan of cool water and heat it slowly—ever so slowly—the frog never registers the level of emergency increasing every so gradually—and allows itself to be cooked.

***

Let's face it—often we spend more waking hours with our colleagues at our place of employment than we do with our families. It feels great to be in supportive work environments where colleagues positively encourage each other and collaborate on projects. An energized, productive place of employment inspires creativity and positivity. It creates a pleasurable energy within a person. What's not to love about colleagues also being great friends?

It can be a very slow, very steady, almost imperceptible slide into hanging out more often, deepening friendship, and a gradual descent into a relationship of intimacy. It happens in such a way that one can't even pinpoint when "the line" was crossed. Affairs often start out with emotional connection. They may never become sexual or perhaps only once the relationship has already become well established. The damage is substantial even if sexual intimacy never occurs.

And while a relationship can start innocently and slide into infidelity without detection, once a person is in an affair, it's brutally difficult to withdraw from that relationship.

Helen Fisher, in her TED talk on The Brain in Love, explains the incredibly powerful pull of love:

> People in love have activity in a tiny factory at the base of the brain... Cells that make dopamine... a natural stimulant... part of the brain's reward system... this is below cognitive thinking, below emotions... part of the reptilian core... associated with wanting, with motivation, with focus and craving. *The same area becomes active when you feel the rush of cocaine.*[xi]

We are acutely aware of the addictive power of cocaine. The motivation and desire for the new hidden relationship is similarly biologically powerful. The craving for the forbidden relationship seems incredible. It seems utterly irresistible to continue contact with the affair partner.

What looks like a choice doesn't actually feel like much of a choice. The pull is extremely compelling.

The challenge is that this is below conscious awareness—out of the realm of rational logic. Science has shown this mighty passion lasts about 18 months in a relationship—any relationship.

A person in an affair can come to the conclusion: "I love my spouse, but I'm not 'in love' with my spouse."

The short term, cocaine-like passion created in the exciting novelty of a new relationship is tough competition for a stable, secure, loving relationship with routines and patterns.

It's a little like choosing between the Corvette convertible and a 4 door mid-size sedan.

Who wouldn't choose the Corvette for an afternoon? I would!! Absolutely!

As a lifestyle, though, my choice is the sedan—every time. How am I going to cart groceries home, drive the kids, be warm in the dead of winter, and many other reasons make the mini-van have much more staying power and be my choice.

Besides, this is an imperfect metaphor—because the Corvette of an affair inevitably morphs into a sedan—and the one from an affair generally doesn't run on all cylinders, and so there is no keeping the corvette.

Relationships begin with the fun of a Corvette convertible—our brains are designed that way. But *they are intended to settle* into a comfortable, useful, secure, solid mid-sized vehicle that will provide the richness of a lifetime of a great ride.

***

One of the most enjoyable parts of my job is working with engaged couples about to get married. They don't come in with relationship problems. They come in because they recognize premarital counseling is a great idea. Premarital counseling is a great proactive way to create a lifelong partnership.

The couples that come for pre-marriage counseling generally come with a solid and good relationship they seek to make even better.

It's inspiring to observe these couples invest in their bond.

They hold hands during sessions, speak warmly and supportively of each other, with each other, and to each other.

And they have no idea that there will probably come a day when they will experience temptation and have to make a choice about whether to stay faithful. Right now, they can't imagine anything other than total devotion to their partner.

I'm not sure I've ever met a partner at the beginning of a relationship that ever plans to be unfaithful.

But it happens. It is thought somewhere between 30-50% of couples will have an episode of cheating where one partner breaks the vows of fidelity. Relationships don't start out with one intending to hurt the other.

It happens. A little tiff has a partner leave in a huff—and then a supportive co-worker asks about the air of upset, and it feels so good to get it off one's chest. And later you're embarrassed to tell your partner you told your supportive co-worker about your fight—and there is a window where a wall should be—and a wall where a window should be.

***

The pre-emptive strike? The way to keep the walls and windows where they should be? Here it is:

Have a discussion about what appropriate walls and windows[xii] look like in your marriage—a checklist of sorts perhaps.

Decide what works for you, and what doesn't work for you as a couple. Determine what each of you are comfortable with, and know ahead of time what is red flag behavior.

An ability to monitor and check your behavior against what you've decided is appropriate behavior can be incredibly helpful. Make those decisions when you are feeling calm and connected with your spouse. Develop the guidelines together. You can use them when you may not be thinking so clearly in the future.

***

Remember the frog in hot water?

What if the frog (assuming frogs can be this smart—work with me—Imaginations please!) jumped out at a set temperature, regardless of how it was feeling?

It would save itself from certain death.

Similarly, it's helpful to have markers you've decided as a couple each of you will not cross.

Now comes the hard part—what to do if/when you pass over that line—*because we know it happens.*

It would be sorely tempting to hide that fact; to avoid telling your partner you did something s/he wouldn't like. The hard part is to "open up the window" to your partner on it. Telling your spouse you crossed a line with another person is brutally challenging, but it is a vote for the marriage—big time.

How very difficult, but productive, to say something like, "I did something today I don't think you'll like. And it's something I'm really not proud of. I had lunch with _____ today…just her and I. I talked about our fight last night…and I regret that. She was so supportive. It felt better to talk to her than is healthy. I'm sorry but I wanted to let you know. Now you know more than she does…and because you are so important, I want you to be the closest one to me."

That repositions the spouse to be the one "in the know" and most intimate with you.

That makes it harder for the walls to get thicker in your marriage and windows to get larger in the illicit relationship.

This is hard, brutally difficult. But it opens a window and lets your partner in. The transparency is admirable.

**

An equally brutal hard part is for the spouse to hear this and work to not only acknowledge the pain, but to **also realize the value of the window** that is being enlarged and maintained in the relationship. It's hard to appreciate a window when the view through it is one that is hurtful. Most often, it will not be heard gratefully. It will be heard with a reaction of hurt. And we know that when people are hurt, they often respond protectively being furious.

To stay grounded and to be grateful for the open discussion rather than to shame and judge for the admission is a difficult—but a worthwhile task, indeed.

It would be very troublesome to hear of a partner's temptation to talk more with a co-worker than necessary, or hear of a new online friend.

In fact, **I can think of few things more challenging**.

**

An actual affair would be one of those things.

Certainly, one of the few things more difficult would be to find out a few months later that your spouse has had an innocent relationship blossom into something that is not at all innocent anymore.

It requires "Big Picture" thinking for these difficult conversations to be successful. It's key to remember that strong marital bonds can hold under the weight challenging conversations. To know your partner finds you safe enough to talk to about even such a painful and complex topic is a *compliment to the relationship* and the spouse.

Odd but true.

An alternate strategy is to have an accountability group. It might even be one individual (who is a same sex person for a heterosexual person) to report and discuss any temptation or difficulties. It is helpful to have one or two people who are committed to being utterly transparent with you and you with them. These would be people with whom you trust and feel safe. People with whom you can share your vulnerabilities and temptations. Talking about it with an accountability partner who is mandated to help you stay faithful to your marriage vows often has the effect of "breaking the spell" of that potential relationship. Knowing that another person will ask you about this relationship at a future meeting assists you in honoring your own values as circumstances unfold.

These friends are assigned the task of helping you stay on the path that ultimately you want to be on. They are pro-marriage/pro-long-term-relationship and supportive of your relationship of your spouse and work to help you keep it strong. This means finding not just buddies who nod and smile, but folks who are willing to challenge you and gently walk alongside you during rough spots. They can say wise and tough things in a way that inspires you to make wise choices when your brain isn't thinking with its smartest parts. Sometimes, a pair or group is created where members do this with and for each other.

This is tough stuff.

To stay faithful in a world that offers temptations as near as a few clicks of a mouse away on online chat rooms is a challenge. It's not always easy to prevent the slippery slide during an intense, marathon project at the office.

These conversations are hard to have, even for couples that are used to having them. They may be impossible to have for couples who have never been this vulnerable and candid with each other before.

This is where a professional can help. A therapist can guide you through these conversations. A counsellor can help create a positive conversation around such a difficult topic. The goal would be to create a stronger bond between you, rather than distance and outrage, as you discuss the issues. Therapy is very helpful to talk about relationships that are seemingly "just friends" but actually feel sinister and threatening.

These conversations are hard, but worthwhile. The reward of a lifelong earned, fought-for, valued, treasured growing marriage makes it worth it.

14 DOES YOUR MARRIAGE NEED A COMA?

Sometimes, a marriage is in such bad shape, it needs a coma.

A Controlled Separation is to a couple, what a Medically Induced Coma is to a severely injured patient.

***

Let me explain:

Scientific American explained Medically Induced Coma in an article.[xiii] A medically induced coma is a state of unconsciousness created using medication. It is only induced by highly trained physicians. It slows the body's metabolism down to allow a swelling brain to heal. The coma protects the brain from further damage that could be caused by further swelling.

Medically induced comas are a drastic measure that attempts to save a life. They are used when the injuries are life threatening.

The article also says that although the medically induced coma is carefully done under the full supervision of doctors with medication, there are risks. There is an effort is made to make the period of coma as brief as possible.

The subtitle to the article: **Medically induced comas are only utilized when other options are lacking.**

In other words, it's a last ditch attempt. And when nothing else is working, a medically induced coma can potentially save a person's life.

Not nearly always.

But sometimes.

***

There are times in some marriages where the relationship is so raw that even attempts to save the marriage create further damage.

Occasions when desperate attempts to fix it are received poorly and make things worse.

Sometimes, the bitter reaction to a relationship crisis catches one or both spouses off guard. Yelling, throwing objects, saying nasty jabs out of character, waking a spouse up in the middle of the night to ask questions for which there are no good answers. A person may feel powerless to stop even though it's clear this isn't helpful. The *collateral damage* forms another whole level of crap to work through.

Other times, a person is going through their own internal turmoil that creates distance within the couple. The pair is having trouble connecting while one spouse is overwhelmed with their own private suffering. It seems too much to work on themselves as an individual and within the marriage. They can't breathe or think or live even one more day like this.

Still other times, the couple has been struggling for eons. Distance. Anger. Disappointment. Disengagement. They can't remember how they got here, they only know it cannot continue. It's bad, it's been bad for a long time...but there are no bad people here.

But there are kids—and calling it quits doesn't appear like an option either.

In these situations, a marriage coma may be just what is needed to stop the damage.

The marriage coma creates an opportunity for:

- Recovery for one or both spouses. People can do their own individual work steadily and solidly without couple dynamics creating complications. When a spouse is in a better place, they are primed to better work on the relationship.
- The collateral damage stops. No more yelling, throwing objects, people saying words that can't be unsaid or unheard. The agony is felt by the individuals, and shared with a therapist or friend, but the marriage isn't frayed by nasty behavior between spouses.
- Sober second thought. To choose to end a marriage that has lasted for years is a gigantic deal. Children are affected. So are in laws. So are retirement plans. Mortgages, friends, traditions, Christmas morning, and family weddings. So much is impacted when a marriage dies.

To decide to end a marriage is a huge decision. Divorce, a decision that will affect you for the rest of your life, is best made calmly from a place of strength, rather than a desperate result to get out of an intolerable situation.

***

A Controlled Separation differs greatly from a "trial" separation. A trial separation is like an experiment to see if singleness works. A trial separation and a Controlled Separation are not the same.

A Controlled Separation is deliberate. It's hard work.

It's a desperate act that says, "We will not give up easily. We are not declaring divorce is inevitable without giving it everything we've got."

It's an opportunity to say: "The marriage we had is over. That wasn't working. Is it possible to get a new and viable marriage to rise out of the ashes?"

A Controlled Separation often recognizes divorce might be on the table, but it slows the process to arrive at a final verdict. Divorce is a big decision. A Controlled Separation allows for sober second thought. It creates a situation where the permanent decision is made from a grounded place.

There are a few basic components of a Controlled Separation. It is best openly discussed and then written down clearly. The written agreement works to remove fear and improve understanding:

1.   A couple figures out how to create that space—renting an apartment, creating an area within the house, one spouse living with family/friends

2.   Negotiate practical matters: looking after the children, finances, etc.

3.   Arrange and agree on appropriate contact with each other. Dating? Therapy? Texting? How much?

4.   Outline the intentional work for each partner. Reading books? Resting? Therapy? Journaling? Retreats? Getting together with friends? Alcoholics Anonymous? What does each person need to grow, heal, and learn?

5.   Establish a time frame.

Lee Raffel writes an excellent book, *Should I Stay or Go? How*

Controlled Separation (CS) Can Save Your Marriage[xiv], that explains the whole process in detail.

***

Some great shifts can happen in a Controlled Separation as there is space for discovery and healing:

- A spouse can realize she isn't bringing her best self to the relationship because of how she pushes herself so hard in every area of her world. She is harder on herself than anyone else. She knows this because she is just as stressed when she is living apart from him, so she starts to work on the way she relates to herself. She begins to talk to her husband differently, once she begins to live a healthier, less stressed life.

- A spouse might understand he hasn't taken initiative to create the marriage he wants. He hasn't told her what works for him. He begins to have conversations where he lets her in on what makes him sad and happy and excited and angry. She loves he is opening up and now doesn't have to guess at what he's thinking.

- A spouse might realize it's the marriage he hates, not the spouse. The patterns in their lives are killing their relationship. Once removed from the day to day destructive systems, the underlying love is perceived. The patterns emerge clearly and can now be addressed and shifted.

- An opportunity to develop empathy. It may be that a spouse can discover the unfair distribution of labor before the separation. Experiencing life in the house with the children and their schedules on their own for a period of time is a revelation. It can be a good thing to experience what it is like to be overwhelmed with responsibilities that normally fall to the other. The spouse understands the other's resentment in a manner previously impossible.

- With the distance created in the separation—not sharing the bed, no obligatory morning pecks, and no evening television together, one has a chance to find the part that misses their spouse. People lose touch for the part of them that feels affection and longing because it has been buried under the anger, that is buried under the fear. The part that loves is too easily buried underneath all of the negative emotion in the every day nattering and nitpicking of life.

Controlled Separation creates capacity for healing, for exploring, for *feeling all the feels* more freely. Sometimes space allows for new hope to emerge. The fragile coals of the relationship can reignite into flames that haven't been around for a while.

To be straightforward, sometimes Controlled Separation leads to growth and clarity that makes divorce the best choice. It can't save a marriage that isn't save-able. There are times the Controlled Separation makes it clear to one or the other that marriage is no longer realistic. But it can save a marriage that might end prematurely because, it feels too painful to stay together in that moment.

***

Insanity: Doing the same thing over and over, expecting different results.

Einstein didn't say it, though many sources say he did. Doesn't matter where it comes from. This much is true: When a marriage is struggling under the weight of:

- regular fights,
- squabbles in predictable and painful patterns,
- agonizing distance,
- excruciating disengagement,

…doing the same thing of hanging in there endlessly doesn't make much sense. The arguments get worse, the patterns deepen, the distance becomes greater, and the disengagement more impenetrable.

The alternative doesn't have to be:

1.   this ugly marriage or

2.   painful divorce.

***

There is a third way. Look for it. Controlled separation. New marriage. New patterns. New ways of relating together.

Stop the hurting. Allow for restoration.

A medically induced coma is a desperate measure to save a patient's life. If a doctor doesn't try it, it would be negligence. Don't we owe our marriages the same opportunity for healing?

Controlled Separation isn't for the faint of heart.

But neither is divorce.

Sometimes, as painful and frightening as it seems, Controlled Separation is a helpful option.

15 DOES YOUR WIFE IMPACT YOUR LIFE?

This chapter gives you language to talk to your husband—take paragraphs of it and write it in your own hand to give to him. Add in your own words that convey the pain in your spirit. Or copy these pages him and put a star beside the bits that express your heart. Highlight the pieces that speak longings of your soul so he can see the parts you need him to know as truth. Heck, hand over this whole letter if you think that'll work best.

This is a direct letter, but it gives a critical message in a civil tone, which isn't always easy when you're tired, angry, and hurt.

Direct is necessary, but it's also vital to phrase your words in a manner that makes them easier to land on him, rather than be pushed away. It's not your duty to "make him listen"—that's his job. It is your responsibility to engage him so he knows this comes from a place inside you that wants to reconnect with him.

This is not a nice letter, but it is deeply kind.

***

Dear husbands-whose-wives-are lonely-for-you,

I'm writing this message to you because I want you to spend the rest of your days with the love of your life. Truly I do. Some of these words may sound harsh, but they are deliberately bold and blunt because the message is so important.

Some of you may recognize yourselves in this letter. Ask your wife how this letter applies to you?

Some of you may have been given a copy of this letter, or it was left on the front seat of your car, or slipped into your laptop case to find. If you are reading this because your spouse gave it to you—do me a favor?

Thank her.

Seriously, yes—thank her.

Let your partner know she was very brave and very kind to give it to you. Let her experience this letter was a lot to digest so you are thanking her, but you won't be able to discuss it further just yet because you need some time to think it through. I know that you want this marriage to work as much as she does—you had no idea how much it wasn't working for her. Implore to her so she will understand that you want to take it seriously and make lasting changes. Mostly let her know you studied it, and it matters to you.

This letter will not be easy to read. It may even make you furious, or want to hide, or get drunk or pull away, or get involved in a super big project in the garage or at work or at the community center to avoid the conversations this letter invites. You may be pissed off because of the implications of this letter.

You may have devoted your life to providing her a wonderful life with secure finances and a beautiful house. You may take her on a big vacation once a year. There are lots of signs you can point to, to show you have really tried to give her what you thought was a a great life. When you receive and read this letter, it will really hurt because all your good intentions won't feel good enough.

Understand I write it because I want you to stay married to the woman of your dreams.

I'm giving you the biggest "heads up" of your life. I'm giving you an opportunity to ensure that your wife isn't slipping away from you unawares.

I'm appealing to you to truly and deeply connect with your wife so she experiences you authentically connecting to her. Being pals and roommates isn't enough. Drawing her into your interests and passions isn't enough.

There may be cues she has given you in the past that invited you to work on your relationship with her. Remember how you have written it off as a cranky mood? Maybe you chalked it up to "that time of the month". Or when she mentioned that the two of you go on the couple's retreat—she alluded to it three times before she dropped it because you said nothing. She suggested you read a book—remember? She even asked you in a joking manner to engage in a quiz or exercise from the internet—she thought perhaps something quick and fun would be a way to invite you to the conversation. What if I told you they were brave bids for connection and when you blew the bids off, she felt blown off?

It's now harder for her to do it again. And so she may not say much.

As the two of you raise your kids, and get together with friends, and buy groceries and pay down the mortgage, and just generally live your lives, she is getting farther and farther away from you. Maybe you haven't even noticed.

Some of these wives wake up one morning and announce, "no

more".

First the bad news: The awful truth that research confirms:

Women initiate divorce 69% of the time.

Yep, over 2/3's of divorces happen because the wife says, "I'm done". There are lots of articles that speculate about why women are more likely to initiate divorce. Look it up on the internet. Yes, I'm asking you to do research. Yes, fuss a little—for the sake of the one you long ago decided to treasure for the rest of your life.

***

Dear husbands-whose-wives-are lonely-for-you,

I will give you my experience of this, from the viewpoint of the therapist's chair. This is harsh but true. I've been doing therapy for years, and the walls of our counseling office have witnessed the same painful story repeatedly:

We get an email or a phone call from a desperate husband (often first thing in the morning). He says his wife wants to end their marriage. He is shocked and stunned. He loves her and wants to continue the marriage. He is distraught. He wants an appointment today. As soon as possible. He will move heaven and earth to be there.

And he's hoping his wife will come too. They simply have to work this out. He's sure they can work it through. She's upset, but things can't really be that bad. He doesn't understand why she wants their marriage to end, because things haven't been that bad. There's gotta be a way to fix this, he believes—as long as she shows up. He really, really wants her to come.

They come in together. He is incredulous and incredibly upset. She is tired and flat. She says in an even tone:

"I've tried for years. I've let him know this isn't working for me. He would get a little more helpful for a few days or weeks, pitching in here and there, but then when I stopped complaining, he would slide back. He would get a little more conversational or affectionate for a few months, and then it drifted back to the way it has always been."

"I can't do this anymore. I believe he wants to change now. I know he thinks it can be different this time. But I'm done. I don't trust the changes he will make now to last. It's too hard to hope he might actually change—I've hoped before and then been disappointed. Can't do it anymore. I'm done."

Sometimes, he comes in alone because she has refused. All of a sudden, he can see crystal clear into their history. In the session, he tells an insightful tale of how he gradually stopped being curious about her interests, how his eyes glazed over when she came home excited from something and she wanted to talk. He can see how he avoided getting up from the couch and let her do most of the house management. He's crushed and desperately motivated to sincerely change—but it's looking like he won't get a chance.

Dear husbands-whose-wives-are lonely-for-you, you don't want that to be you, do you?

***

A wife will advise me she endeavored to reach out to you and has been disappointed for as long as she can remember. She has worked to be:

- supportive of your career with late evenings at work by taking over tasks at home,
- a cheerleader for you as you pursue your interests while you went away for the weekend or spent money on your latest pursuit, and

112

- patient with your fatigue and let you go to bed early while she made the lunches and got ready for the next day. (Were you even aware of how tired she was?)

She has devoted years to:

- tolerate your disengagement
- silently enduring your lack of interest and support in her life
- compensate for your distance with the kids and create excuses for you

A wife often does a lot to make her husband's life easier without him realizing it. This might mean giving up her own opportunities to be with her friends. Or compromising her career or interests in ways she wouldn't even have brought up to you. Or even just making your favorite suppers often and rarely making hers.

Statistically, she has done a lot more housework than you have. She has learned to not raise the issue; you taught her it would only lead to a fight. She has just silently been working more hours than you in a day because everyone expects it.

More than likely, she has gone for pizza when you wanted pizza, or burgers when you wanted burgers. Have you invested in discovering which new little bistro interests her that she is hoping to try? When is the last time you want to a restaurant she liked that you're not really nuts about, but you went because you knew she'd love it? And then she saw that you truly enjoyed the experience of going to her restaurant because you got to see the sparkle of delight in her eye.

***

There are a lot of women who are unhappy, but are determined to be kind and respectful. She knows whining and complaining doesn't draw a husband into a closer marriage.

So she tells her husband that something isn't right and she would like to go for counseling. When the husband refuses, she doesn't know what else to say. So she says nothing. Her silence is nice and robs you of the truth. Giving you the unpopular reality would actually be kind.

Your disappointed wife may leave a marriage book on the coffee table or the nightstand for a looooong time, hoping you'll notice and pick it up, because she intuitively knows you, for sure, will not read it if she asks you directly. She may have even highlighted certain passages she is desperate to have you digest—and you walk by the book every day without acknowledgement.

There is distance you feel from her. Less sex. Maybe no sex at all. For quite a while. You notice and mention it because you miss it. But you tune out when she tries to tell you of the distance she feels.

And so when you rebuffed her direct and indirect efforts, she gave up and hung in there, enduring her existence in your marriage for as long as she could.

And then one day, she writes a letter and packs a suitcase, saying she's done.

Women tend to file for divorce when they are done.

Finished. Finito. So very, very done.

***

Dear Husband-whose-wife-is-lonely-for you—don't let this be your wife. Please.

The wife will use the counseling session he now suddenly dragged her to, to explain that there is nothing left in her to work on this marriage. Leaving now is like when the doctor declares the time of death over a patient.

She isn't killing the marriage—she's acknowledging it is already dead.

Typically, husbands-whose-wives-are lonely-for-you, only now is when the husband gets it is truly serious. And all the feelings of love and adoration flood him. He truly loves his wife.

And he is desperate to fix it. He doesn't want to lose her.

Except she's done.

So, dear husbands-whose-wives-are lonely-for-you, I realize you don't mean harm to your wife. You don't mean to allow the marriage to die in front of you without you even knowing about it. You don't mean to ignore her. I get that.

It's not intentional.

It's hard to hear from your life partner she finds you falling short. It's tempting to push painful and distasteful information away, like pushing away the Brussel sprouts on your plate and just not eating them.

Women are raised to be sensitive to other's emotions…they recognize when their husband is upset and take care of it. They perceive when he needs extra support, and they give it. Wives really dial in to being mindful of where their partners are at—what their preferences and desires are, what their interests are, what bothers and irritates them, and what has them laugh with joy. Women are socialized to be acutely aware of and be impacted by other individuals in their lives.

So, husbands-whose-wives-are lonely-for-you, this is hard stuff. It's quite possible you weren't raised in our culture to accept influence.

You haven't grown up in a climate where it was your task to figure out how to actually have what your wife is feeling matter to you in ways that have you check in on her. It perhaps will not occur to you to postpone the time you go on your fishing trip to fit into her day, or offer to take over cleaning up the house because you see she's tired, or learn to watch some of her movies the way she may have learned to watch yours.

Simply put:

Does your wife experience and see by your actions and your words that her feelings, thoughts and behaviors influence you? Does she see you living a life that actively demonstrates she matters to you?

To accept influence from their husbands is as natural as breathing to most wives.

For most men, accepting influence from their wives doesn't come as naturally.

And accepting influence from your wife, according to John Gottman, one of the leading researchers of love, is critically important in reducing your risk of divorce.[xv]

So, husbands, there is a brief inventory online that can get you thinking about how well you accept your wife's influence. You can find it here: <https://www.gottman.com/blog/weekend-homework-assignment-do-you-and-your-partner-accept-each-others-influence/>[xvi]

Take it—and take the results sincerely.

Better yet, when you've had a chance to gather yourself to truly listen to her, ask your wife how much she feels like she matters to you. Ask her how much she feels heard and understood, how much she feels you support and care for her. That will be hard. It will take real courage.

I'm warning you—if she has given you this letter, either in the book or printed it a version of it out, the results may be dismal. That will certainly be disheartening. You may unleash the flood gates of pain.

Her parched soul is so thirsty for connection it may overwhelm you. Your first impulse perhaps will be to become angry. You might want to blame her. Can you prepare yourself to hold off on a harsh reaction?

The irony is that, even in the gentle asking of what's behind this letter, you are telling her she matters. When you listen to her and give her an experience of listening to her responses that encourages her to say even more hard stuff to you, she feels valued. If you can keep her talking, and if you can write stuff down, and really hear her—as hard as it will be—it will be an important step in letting her know that she can feel hope.

It will seem strange to let her talk and open up about her frustration, anger, heartbreak and loneliness while just saying, "I want to know more. I didn't know, and thank you now for telling me." Don't fix anything. Don't try explaining. It is not the time for explanations or repair—the irony in this is that as you simply hold her pain, the repair has already begun.

**

Dear husbands-whose-wives-are-lonely-for-you, get an accurate read from her on your marriage, now, before she tells you so clearly that there is nothing you can do about it.

Please?

I want you to be able to grow old and happy with your wife.

Make my job as a therapist easier? If she asks you to work on your marriage now before she is completely burnt out—please show up?

Stick with the process—and you give yourself a fighting chance?

You give your therapist something to work with when you come before your wife is completely done.

16 A LETTER TO POTENTIAL CLIENTS: YEP, THERAPY IS HARD

Whether or not your husband is willing to go to therapy, you may benefit from going to counseling, even if it is alone. It's a chance to learn about yourself, your input into the marriage, and how where you come from shapes your responses to him. Consider counseling for yourself as a wife whose marriage is needs some work.

***

If your husband will consider counseling, then pass this on to him?

***

Hey, if you're reading this, it's because your wife has said the two of you need therapy. It may have come as a calm request. Or maybe a gentle plea.

Or the two of you may be past all that and you're reading because of an ultimatum: Show up to couple therapy with me or we're done.

I suspect you've avoided marriage counseling in the past because the whole idea seems foreign to you. Distasteful.

Too touchy-feely.

I'll give you that.

Yep, therapy often does involve talking about feelings.

However, think back to the beginning of your relationship. Did you get married merely because it seemed the practical and logical thing to do? Remember the powerful and passionate feelings that drove you to decide to spend the rest of your lives together?

And trust me, it is your feelings right now have you resist therapy. The very thing that could save and enrich the most important relationship is something that raises discomfort and unease inside. It is feelings that have kept you out of the therapy room.

Feelings are important. As inconvenient as it may be, feelings drive behavior.

You've heard your spouse and are now considering therapy. Let me talk to you about what therapy is about. It might surprise you.

***

My husband, Jim, and I made a deal with each other when we got married. We promised one another if either one of us said to the other: "I'd like to go talk to a therapist," the other will agree to go. No excuses or wiggling out.

The idea is that if one of us feels like we need to go to a counselor, it's quite possible it is because the other is feeling misunderstood or not heard in the relationship. And if that is the case, it would be quite possible the very reason why therapy is perceived to be needed by one of us couldn't be understood by the other.

Do you know your own blind spots? Of course not! Nobody, by definition, can recognize their own blind spots.

Jim and I talk regularly about how each of us is feeling in our relationship. I would love to be aware if Jim, for some reason, starts to feel like something isn't right. If his attempts to describe it to me about it don't go well, I actually do want to know. I want him to have a way to address it. Part of loving Jim is ensuring that our marriage is serving him well.

I'm acutely aware I'm not perfect. So, I may not only flub up, but then also botch the way I handle it when he tries to tell me about my goof. Our marriage only works well if it is working for both of us. If it isn't working for him, then it's not working for me either.

***

I'd like you to be aware of a few things you need to appreciate as a person who is contemplating counseling. Many consider the idea of therapy only as a passing fancy, meant for other people. Many potential clients wonder about making an appointment, maybe even want an appointment. But they don't ever attend therapy.

I want to ensure that if you decide to not come to counseling, you are doing it for the right reasons.

I spoke to a friend this week who is in serious crisis. Other friends of ours were encouraging her to make an appointment with a therapist. In the end she spent the money given to her for a session on paint for her bedroom. She spent her spare time for a week making her bedroom into her own little personal haven—a beautiful place to rest when the world feels harsh and confusing. She maintains that this was the best therapy for her.

Good on her for making that decision!

She did some important healing. She did therapy. She gave her soul some nourishing healing, just not by chatting with a therapist while sitting in a love seat in an office with a therapist.

Sometimes a new coat of paint truly is therapy.

Go for it...or any other activities/relationships that are truly healing. Grab real healing wherever you can get it.

But sometimes people who don't attend therapy avoid healing altogether.

That makes me sad.

***

It's hard for some folks to really know there might be healing from the hurting. There are always reasons they aren't grabbing the opportunity, and squeezing it.

I love when people seize an opportunity to heal. Whether it is painting the walls of their room, or therapy—take healing opportunities and squeeze them like the gift they are. Be meticulously careful to squeeze every last drop of healing out of the opportunity into your heart.

It's vital to explore the underlying reasons people choose to not go to counseling for healing. I'm going to invite you to ponder on these. Decide if you are choosing not to go to counseling for valid reasons. These are common reasons that I think are powerfully and strongly given for not going to counseling, that in my mind, just don't hold up:

1. You've been told counseling is for sissies (or wimps, or weaklings or something of the sort)

Evidently you've never witnessed a counseling session.

Simply put: therapy is one long exercise in vulnerability.

Brené Brown, one of my favorite researchers, says that vulnerability sounds like truth and feels like courage. But it is never weakness. I see it be true.

My clients show me raw courage. Every. Single. Day.

***

Therapy is hard and risky work. It means:

- Going to places long buried deep inside and saying things out loud that haven't seen the light of day for years, or perhaps ever.
- Acknowledging your own responsibility for the way you have said or done (or not said or done) that have contributed to struggles and distance in your marriage.
- Expressing discomfort about your troublesome marriage with a therapist...and then even to your wife.
- Being real about how fears that have developed from the ghost of trauma past continue to pull the strings in your life.
- Going beneath the anger to acknowledge the fear, or be candid about the loss, or to feel the hurt
- Acknowledging the use of familiar patterns that worked well when you were younger, but now are pulling you out of your authenticity. These old patterns are making it hard for you to show up in your life right now.

Please know if you show up in our therapy offices, you are seen as a person who is strong and courageous in being willing to look at the hardest parts of your life.

I see you, as a new client, as a wise investor.

You are prepared to do complicated things because you believe

123

that the healing inside yourself and in your relationships will be a payoff that is well worth it.

I respect that.

2. You've been told that therapy is all about blaming your mother/father/bully/abuser and it just seems like that's a lousy use of money

Bad things happen to good people. Life isn't fair. Trauma shapes us powerfully. We don't have to like it. It's just truth.

But healing means taking responsibility for your own internal suffering. It means being aware not only of what happened, but how you tell yourself a story about what happened. It means growing to accept that others are often doing the best they can, even when they are doing bad and hurtful things.

Those insights--when you get them at a soul level—well, that changes a person.

It means drawing boundaries and having hard conversations. It means grieving events that will never happen. Letting go of the dreams that will never be. Releasing resentments created by demanding things that are not within a person's capacity.

I'll warn you. Therapy is hard.

Once you start counseling, you won't be able to keep on blaming others for your internal discomfort.

It means looking inside for how your reaction to what has happened shapes your experience of what happened. It's often the story we tell ourselves about what happened that shapes how we see the world. The story we tell ourselves is often an unconscious confabulation where we honestly believe a lie about ourselves or the world.

There is no way to know when we are making up or adding to the data without someone hearing our story and helping us work through it. Perspective is essential...and how are we supposed to see parts of ourselves we can't see?

Pain is inevitable. Suffering is optional.

But trust me—easier said than done.

3. You think it's better to do this alone

For centuries, people believed the earth was flat. Even when science said the world was round, folks denied it, and maintained the belief that the earth was a pancake.

They can believe the earth is a giant Frisbee, but that doesn't change the reality. The earth is a giant ball.

And folks—we are wired for connection. We need each other. Science is very clear on this.

"I don't need anybody" or "I don't let anybody in" or "I'll only get hurt if I am vulnerable" are all emotional and relational equivalents of, "the world is flat".

We understand the world and ourselves best in community. Therapy is an excellent place to start connecting if you live in a world where you have always believed, "I don't need anybody".

I've had folks (most often they are men) tell me within the first 10-15 minutes of a session they have told me more of their inner world than they have told anybody. Ever.

And folks, those people who are opening up--for the first time in their lives—they are terrified and second guessing themselves.

They also *wonder out why they waited so long.* Once people start the process of hearing themselves think out loud with another person, they recognize its value. It's hard and challenging and valuable.

We can't promise you a straight upward line of linear progress. But talking to another person about the secrets and the fears and the inadequacies of one's life paradoxically feels life-giving and soul-saving. It acts like a glass of clean, cool water to a parched and thirsty soul. The dry cracks start to fill in, even in just the sharing of one's story.

It's not only terrifying—it's fantastic!

***

Secrets kill.

Therapy is a great place to start speaking out, to practice talking about the things that secretly hijack your life. Once they are spoken of, they lose their power.

Wayne Brady, a comedian speaks of the tremendous pressure that culture puts on people--especially men--to pretend they are OK, even if they are not OK. He has a great video that can help you understand the pressure.[xvii]

He invites you to consider giving yourself permission to let somebody in.

***

So, dear-person-who-is-considering-counseling, know that we are ready to rumble with you. Make the call or write the email, and get the reckoning started. Get your brave on, and tell your story to someone who wants to help you write a better story.

Perhaps you have some questions about what it is like to book an appointment, or what to expect the first session. Ask whatever you need to, to make it possible for you to show up at an appointment.

You don't have to go to counseling if it's not right for you. But please make sure that you're not just making excuses. Please be candid with yourself if you are avoiding something big in your life.

And if you decide to attend a session alone, or with your spouse, know a few things:

- It's extremely common to notice yourself checking for a sore throat. The day of the appointment, it's quite possible you will think it completely necessary to schedule an emergency meeting for something on the back burner for months. You may suddenly feel a lot of pressure to do something else at the precise time the therapy appointment is scheduled. That's normal. Notice your desire to not attend the session, and store it away as valuable information. Talk to the therapist about your reluctance, if you dare. Still go. Attend the appointment.

- The first session is often an opportunity the therapist has to get the picture of your relationship. Your marriage didn't start to struggle within a day—it's not reasonable to expect huge changes after a single session. Feeling like nothing was fixed within the first session is not a valid reason to stop going. Keep at it for several sessions before you decide.

- Therapy is opening things up; it's creating dialogue where there hasn't been any. If you get angry or scared or upset or feeling blamed, it is because you and your wife are finally talking about something important. Those feelings are uncomfortable, but they aren't information that actually says, "Stop going". Please mention these feelings in session as you go through therapy.

- Therapy is for both of you. It would be weird if you didn't hear things that are painful. When your wife says she is angry about something that you've done, hear it and be curious. Notice when you are upset, but work to hold your discomfort and keep listening. That won't be easy, but it will tell your wife that you find her thoughts and feelings important. You don't have to agree with them, but I will ask you to work towards understanding where they come from. The understanding is far more important to healing the relationship than if you agree with what she is saying. Listen with your heart, not your head. Work to make it right. That's far more important than being right.

- If the therapist ticks you off, tell him/her. That is important. You are important in therapy, just as your spouse is. If something is said that feels inaccurate or painful, bring it up so it can be unpacked and processed. The therapist will not take "sides". The therapist works to help you reach your goals.

- If, after several sessions, it doesn't feel like it is going anywhere, talk with your therapist about it. If you're going together, talk with your spouse about it. Is it because you are resistant to the process, or because the therapist isn't "synching" with you? It absolutely is hard to start with another therapist if the first one doesn't connect with you. But, do recognize that starting with another therapist is not nearly as difficult as a divorce.

- If you don't understand what the therapist means, or what your spouse is saying, just say so. Sometimes we use the same words in different ways. Not understanding and saying so shows your strength and security in yourself.

No matter what, going to a marriage therapist, and sticking with it, shows your wife you are sincere in wanting to make the marriage one that you both enjoy. Therapy might not be easy or pleasant, but most important and good things in our lives that we achieve are borne out of struggle.

I wish you well as you work to improve your marriage!

AFTERWORD

This is not the end.

This is the beginning.

The beginning of hard conversations and wise decision making.

The beginning of making the difficult and messy happen, because if your marriage is already stressed, what do you have to lose?

The beginning of letting go of *nice* and embracing *kind*.

The beginning of remembering your own worth and value as a human being. Of knowing that you are deserving of respect and dignity. That is without question.

The beginning of not settling for something that doesn't work.

The beginning of pursuing the connection that you once had so long ago, you almost can't remember. But it **was** there, long ago.

The beginning of courageous acts that might not be popular, but are deeply and profoundly good.

The beginning of brave utterances that give your spouse the chance to hear your voice, your dreams, your boundaries, your passions, and your desires.

***

It's hard to start, but being heard is ultimately always a good thing. Listening deeply is profound. Always.

I wish you well. I wish you courage and strength as you negotiate difficult circumstances. I wish you laughter and a sense of humor as you reconnect with your love. I wish you wisdom as you decide when and where and how to make your position clear. I wish you discernment as you figure your unique path forward.

ABOUT THE AUTHOR

Carolyn Klassen is director and therapist at Conexus Counselling, a large, respected and busy private practice in Manitoba, Canada.

She has appeared in HuffingtonPost Canada articles and Sun Media national columns, and is a regular weekly guest on one of Canada's flagship talk radio programs, as well as various other media interviews on radio, television, and print.

Carolyn is a dynamic speaker delivering workshops, retreats, and seminars to help people connect more effectively with themselves, others, and The Divine. She writes a blog entitled, "A Thoughtful Look at Life" at <conexuscounselling.ca/blog/>.

Carolyn believes we are wired for connection, giving a 2018 TEDx Winnipeg talk entitled, *Learning from the Sequoias: the Value of Interconnectedness*. She has a special interest in removing barriers that stop people from reaching their goals.

Live the life and have the connections you were created for!

ENDNOTES

i Dr. Michael Rosenfeld from Stanford University has done this research. You can read about it in multiple places, but here is a good place to start:

Robb, A. (2015, August 24) *Why women are more likely than men to initiate divorce.* Retrieved from:
http://nytlive.nytimes.com/womenintheworld/2015/08/24/why-women-are-more-likely-than-men-to-initiate-a-divorce/

ii Bureau of Labor Statistics. (2016, December 20) *American Time Use Survey.* Retrieved from:
https://www.bls.gov/tus/charts/household.htm

iii Benson, K. (2016, October 7*) Emotionally Intelligent Husbands Are Key to a Lasting Marriage.* Retrieved from:
https://www.gottman.com/blog/emotionally-intelligent-husbands-key-lasting-marriage/

iv There are a lot of articles written about Dr. Ronald Rogge's work at the University of Rochester looking at the value of watching and discussing movies as a couple. Solid research that says watching and then discussing the movie reduces divorce rate. See, for example,

Carrol, L. (2014, February 10) *Movie therapy: 8 films that might save your troubled marriage.* Retrieved from:

https://www.today.com/health/movie-therapy-8-films-might-save-your-troubled-marriage-2D12074340

ᵛ I can't recommend Brené Brown's books enough. Daring Greatly in particular is about figuring out how to show up and really dare to be real in your life. This quote is from page 51.

Brown, B. (2015). *Daring Greatly: How the Courage to Be Vulnerable Transforms the Way We Live, Love, Parent, and Lead.* New York: Avery.

ᵛⁱ Another great quote from *Daring Greatly*, page 52.

ᵛⁱⁱ Dr. Sue Johnson has developed Emotionally Focused Couple Therapy (EFT), a model of couple therapy that has some great research behind it. Her books are great ones for couples to read. There are therapists that are knowledgeable in her approach who carefully work with couples on the bond they have with each other. EFT is a model that specifically looks at connection.

The quote is from her website:

Johnson, S. (2017). *A Quiet Revolution.* Retrieved from: http://www.drsuejohnson.com/love/a-quiet-revolution/

ᵛⁱⁱⁱ Klassen, C. (2018, June). *Learning from the Sequoias: the Value of Interconnectedness.* Retrieved from: https://youtu.be/S9BJjkijb2I

ⁱˣ Dr. Sue Johnson created the idea of A.R.E. and it is a key concept in Emotionally Focused Couple Therapy. You can read lots more about it here:

Johnson, S. (2008). *Hold me Tight: Seven Conversations for a lifetime of Love.* New York: Little, Brown and Company.

For a helpful quiz to further think this through between you and your husband, look here:

Adamson, S. (2015, September 9). *How emotionally responsive is your partner?* Dr. Sue Johnson's A.R.E. Questionnaire. Retrieved from:

https://cmfcdallas.com/2015/09/a-r-e-questionnaire/

[x] Lisitsa, Ellie. *The Sound Relationship House: Build Love Maps.* Retrieved from https://www.gottman.com/blog/the-sound-relationship-house-build-love-maps/

[xi] Fisher, H. (Speaker) (2008, February) *The brain in love.* (TED talk) United States: TED.

[xii] Shirley Glass writes eloquently about "walls and windows" in her book looking at infidelity:

Glass, Shirley et al. (2004). *Not "Just Friends": Rebuilding Trust and Recovering Your Sanity After Infidelity.* New York: Atria Books.

[xiii] Biello, D. (2011, January 10). *What is a Medically Induced Coma and Why Is It Used?* Retrieved from: https://www.scientificamerican.com/article/what-is-a-medically-induced-coma/

[xiv] Raffel, L. (1999), *Should I Stay or Go? How Controlled Separation (CS) Can Save Your Marriage.* New York: McGraw Hill.

[xv] Pincus, J. (2017, July 31). *Husbands Can Only Be Influential if They Accept Influence.* Retrieved from: https://www.gottman.com/blog/husband-can-influential-accept-influence/

[xvi] This is meant to start a discussion and raise awareness…not give you a score that is the final judgement of your ability to be a husband:

Lisitsa, E. (No Date). *Weekend Homework Assignment: Do You and Your Partner Accept Each Other's Influence?* Retrieved from:

https://www.gottman.com/blog/weekend-homework-assignment-do-you-and-your-partner-accept-each-others-influence/

[xvii] Brady, W. (2015, January 21). #*StrongerThanStigma* - Wayne Brady: Why I Waited to Talk About My Depression. Retrieved from: https://www.youtube.com/watch?v=KFnwJg_4uwM1